Mindfulness

More Than Just Mindfulness

By: Frank Lin

Table of Contents

Introduction

Mindfulness is a powerful practice that can change your life. The ideology behind mindfulness is rather simple: by achieving a deeper sense of self-awareness, you open yourself up to the ability to have a greater control over yourself and thus over your life in general. However, mindfulness can be a lot deeper than that. And, in reality, a lot harder, too. Many people struggle to attain mindfulness in their life because they attempt to accomplish it all at once. Or, because they fail to understand what mindfulness truly is.

In Buddhist teachings, mindfulness is one of the most important lessons a person can learn. It is the foundation for all of the other teachings that are associated with Buddhism. When reading this book, it is important that you realize that despite the frequent referencing to Buddhism, you are not expected to nor do you have to become a Buddhist in order to use the information within' and enrich your life with it all. You should regard Buddhism as more of a way of life instead of a religion, as this may help you feel more confident and empowered when you are enforcing these new ways of being into your own life.

Remember, you cannot achieve every teaching of mindfulness in a single day. Knowing that, you should take your time when reading this book. Each chapter has been created to help you consider different elements of mindfulness and life, and to help you dive deeper into your own existence and mind. You are not expected to complete this book in one or even two sittings and then suddenly be a mindfulness master. Instead, you should take your time, consider each of the teachings, and then recognize what you can learn within' your own life through those teachings. The slower you take things, the easier it will be for you to grasp this new way of living and enlist it in your own life. Then, you truly will be able to master the art of mindfulness and have utmost control over your entire existence. Please, take your time and enjoy your reading experience!

Part 1: Insight

Mindfulness is a practice that has long been used to help individuals create the state of mind that they really desire: happiness. In Buddhism and Dharma, we learn teachings that guide us to the true meaning of mindfulness, and help us gain clarity on what we must do to become mindful within' ourselves.

Throughout this section, you are going to learn valuable information about what exactly mindfulness is and how valuable it can be in your life. You will also learn about the power of intention and how it can enhance your mindfulness state and lead you into a state of existence that allows you to lead the happy and peaceful life you desire.

Mindfulness isn't easy if you try and start too much all at once, but you can take your time and lead yourself into mindfulness with practical strategies that will guide you there. Then, you will find yourself leading a life that will come from a state of consciousness that allows you to create your life exactly as you desire it to be.

"Mindfulness is simply being aware of what is happening right now without wishing it were different; enjoying the pleasant without holding on when it changes (which it will); being with the unpleasant without fearing it will always be this way (which it won't)."

-James Baraz

Chapter 1: The Value of Mindfulness

Mindfulness has a strong impact on your ability to transform your life and get all that you desire from it. When you are mindful, you open yourself up to the ability to make the internal changes that are necessary for you to acquire the external changes that you desire. Although it appears to be a very spiritual practice, mindfulness is actually a very logical and strategic practice that enables you to unlock many opportunities in life.

Mindfulness is brought up in many areas of life, both spiritual and nonspiritual. You may realize that many extremely successful people, including most billionaires, have included mindfulness into their life. That is because when you are mindful, you are highly focused on what you want in your life and therefore you make decisions that only assist you in attracting those things into your life, nothing else. Often times when we don't practice mindfulness, we end up making decisions that are not focused on our inner most wants, desires and needs. As a result, we end up not having what it is that we want in life because we have not been mindful about our actions in attracting it.

In the past when you have made decisions that you deemed were wrong, you likely realize now that at the time, you had been acting out of emotion. The most common emotion we react from, instead of respond from, is stress. When we are stressed out we act with emotion in a way that is not clearly aimed towards our specific wants or needs in life. Because of this, we may end up actually pushing away what we want and need, instead of drawing it in closer.

Throughout this book, you are going to see a lot of references to Buddhism and Dharma. These teachings offer powerful insights into the way of life and how you can lead a mindful and happy life in general. It is important to realize that these teachings are not exactly a religion, but rather a way of life. Buddhism and Dharma teachings offer a perspective-based study on life without you necessarily having to worship any Gods. As Albert Einstein said: "If there is any religion that could correspond to the needs of modern science, it would be Buddhism."

As you read this book you are going to learn about many ways that you can use mindfulness in your life and how it can powerfully transform your life as a result of your actions. You should make sure that you keep an open mind throughout this process. As much as it may seem so, mindfulness is actually as much practical and logical as it is spiritual. Because of that, you do not necessarily need to be a spiritual or religious person in any way, shape or form in order to use mindfulness and benefit from all that it has to offer.

If you have been struggling to practice mindfulness up until now, it may be because you are leading a lifestyle or carrying habits that present as obstacles to the process of mindfulness. Many times, we have a lifestyle that keeps us reacting out of emotion or simply carrying out mindless activities based on old routines and habits we have built into our lives. These old outdated habits and routines can actually deviate away from our ability to be mindful and our ability to gain value from mindfulness itself. It is important that you learn to start recognizing these obstacles and pay attention so you can find out exactly how you can overcome them and carry on in your mindfulness journey.

When you lead a mindful life, there is so much more to it than just being in a Zen state or doing meditation on a regular basis. Mindfulness is a mental state that you achieve and balance throughout your life as a means to remove as much emotional baggage as you possibly can so that you can free yourself from it. As a result of this freeing activity, you open yourself up to the ability to have an extremely clear mind that will allow you to make every decision and action thoughtfully, instead of acting in reaction to thoughts, emotions or fleeting feelings that you experience.

Knowing that mindfulness is a state of mind that you must achieve and balance, it may become overwhelming to you. This is especially true if you try to achieve mindfulness all in one go, as it can take a lot of work to achieve it. For some, it is even impossible to achieve a mindful state all in one go. The best way for you to do it is to take your time and start becoming mindful of a few things at a time, and working your way up to a totally mindful state of life. For those who try to go too fast, you may discover that it is too hard to face and let go of that much emotional baggage at once, and you may end up feeling worse off as a result. It is best to take your time and focus on what matters most and then work your way up from there.

If you are a more logical based mind, it may help you to understand that Buddhism and Dharma teachings are the best scientific way for human psychology and emotional behavior to be explained to the average person. Through these teachings, you can learn why humans take certain positive or negative psychological and physical based actions and reactions to certain triggers. While the messages can sometimes seem cryptic, they are often easily translatable into something that will allow you to take a realistic and honest look at yourself and apply it in a practical way that will allow you to get closer to the state of total mindfulness.

Chapter Summary:

- Mindfulness is a state of mind that can help you transform your life
- When you are mindful, you are not operating from an emotional state
- Keeping an open mind about this book will help you gain maximum value
- Buddhism and Dharma offer the best teachings about mindfulness
- Buddhism and Dharma are a way of life
- You cannot achieve a mindful state all at once

Chapter 2: Mindfulness Is...

After learning about how powerful mindfulness can be in your life, you are probably wondering what it is exactly and how you can achieve this state. You may be wondering exactly how mindfulness can add all that value to your life, and what it takes to get there. After all, inner peace is what we are all looking for, isn't it?

"Mindfulness practice means that we commit fully in each moment to be present; inviting ourselves to interface with this moment in full awareness, with the intention to embody it as best we can an orientation of calmness, mindfulness, and equanimity right here and right now."

-Jon Kabat-Zinn

Mindfulness is a state of consciousness, if you are looking for the most basic definition. However, if you want to get deeper into it, the practice of mindfulness means you are paying attention "on purpose". You are purposefully and consciously directing your awareness, instead of allowing your awareness to ride on "autopilot". It is important to realize that mindfulness and awareness are two separate words, and that although they are often interchanged, they are actually two separate things. It is best if you learn to separate them now and that you do not get into the habit of using these words interchangeably.

Self-awareness involves a vague awareness of your current state from moment to moment. For example, you may be aware that you are feeling angry. However, that is not the same as being mindful about your anger. If you were being mindful about your anger, you would be purposefully aware of the anger, meaning that you would notice every element of it. Instead of just realizing you were angry, you would realize every element of your anger and how it was affecting you. You would recognize what is happening around you that is triggering this anger, and you would recognize the internal state that it is bringing up.

Let's take a look at the practice of drinking tea to further explore what mindfulness is and how you can be mindful. Imagine you are drinking a tea in the mid-afternoon. At this time, you are likely also thinking about what is on the television, something you heard about earlier today, and several other things all at the same time as you are drinking your tea. You may be aware of the tea, and you may even be aware of the unique flavor, but you are not being mindful about the experience of drinking the tea. In this circumstance, you are likely only vaguely aware of your experience of drinking the tea in your cup, and potentially some of the sensations involved. It is likely, however, that you are not aware of the thoughts and emotions attached with that beverage.

This occurs because, in our natural state, we are only vaguely aware of our thoughts as they occur. Our thoughts often wander about from thought to thought in an unrestricted manner. When we are being mindful, though, our thoughts will remain on what we are doing in the present moment. We will be less focused on what happened in the past or what we expect to or hope will happen in the future and more focused on what is happening in the present moment. We will think about the situation we are in, the environment around us, the feelings we are having, and all of the senses that are being awakened and used throughout the experience.

The part of mindfulness that is the most important part is the purposefulness of it. When you are living with the purpose of staying in the same space as your present moment, whether you are staying in tune with a particular emotion or physical experience, this means that you are actively taking control over your mind and shaping it with your own intention.

"Mindfulness isn't difficult; we just need to remember to do it."

-Sharon Salzberg

When it is left to its own devices, your mind will take the time to wander through all sorts of thoughts. These thoughts express all different types of emotions from sadness, anger, revenge, depression, happiness, joy and otherwise. The more that you allow yourself to indulge in these thoughts, the more you reinforce those emotions within' your own heart and cause yourself to suffer. The majority of the time when we are suffering from our thoughts, we are remembering events that happened in the past that caused painful emotions in us. It is important that we take the time to realize that the past is over and no longer exists. The only moment that we can actually experience is the present moment, and this seems to be the one that we often do our best to avoid, usually through thoughts and emotions.

As you can see, mindfulness is purposefully being present in the moment and noticing exactly what is happening right now, not before and not after. Knowing this, it doesn't mean that we cannot think about the past or the future. However, when we do, we should ensure that we are doing so from a mindful state of consciousness that allows us to stay aware that we are not currently existing in that time and the only moment we have is the present. Therefore, we can choose how we will consciously allow for that experience to change us or affect us.

There are many ways that you can learn to become present in the moment. Later in this book, you will learn about practical methods to achieving mindfulness. These tools are a great way for you to successfully exit an emotionally charged state of mind that may be causing you to suffer and will allow for you to use your state of consciousness to grow. When you purposefully direct your awareness, you are able to "anchor" yourself in the present experience and decrease the effect that certain thoughts and emotions can have on your life. Instead, you will be able to create a space of freedom where you can allow calmness and contentment to grow.

Chapter Summary:

- Mindfulness is a state of peace, not necessarily happiness
- Self-Awareness and mindfulness are two different things
- Mindfulness is being purposefully aware of yourself
- Our mind wanders if we don't consciously choose our thoughts
- Mindfulness is being present in the moment you're in
- You can still think about the past and future, just do so mindfully

Chapter 3: The Intention

In the previous chapter, you learned about the importance of intention when you are being mindful. Intention and purpose define the difference between mindfulness and simply being in a state of awareness. Initially, mindfulness is hard. You will not be able to achieve it all at once, and it may take many months or even years to become mindful in all areas of your life. As you practice these new patterns and intentions, however, you will find that it becomes more instinctual for you to become mindful in your everyday life.

"Your life is like a fish in a drying well, what's to rejoice?"

– Frank Lin

The above quote emphasizes that we are all here with a limited amount of time to be around. We only get so many journeys around the sun before we expire. Knowing that, there is no sense in making one moment more special than the next. Instead, we should do our best to be purposefully mindful of all moments and find peace and happiness in them as much as we possibly can. Like the fish in the drying well, we are destined to die, and therefore why would we waste our time putting any single moment on a pedestal over the rest? Whether the moments you hold dear are ones that have passed or ones that are yet to come, it is best to acknowledge them for what they truly are: moments that no longer exist. There is no purpose in letting yourself use these moments as a means to suffer. Instead, acknowledge them and then bring yourself back to the present moment as much as you possibly can. Eventually, it will become easy to do so.

When you are seeking to live in a mindful state, you should realize that you aren't actually seeking to live in a constant state of happiness. That in itself would draw away from your happy experiences and dilute their value in your life. Instead, mindfulness is the practice of living a more peaceful existence. When you live this way, you will result in having heightened levels of success in multiple areas of your business because you are able to think objectively and thus make objective decisions in your life. This mindset allows you to eliminate the actions we take as a result of emotional baggage as allows you to think more clearly and make decisions that will have a more positive result on your success in life overall. This success will be experienced not in just one area of your life, but in all.

When you are mindful, you may feel as though you are living in a state of delayed gratification. In this day and age, we are all about instant gratification and often find ourselves reacting to everything from an emotional state of mind. As a result, many of our actions are emotionally charged and are not done with our highest benefit in mind. This is the case when we are not living in a state of mindfulness. Oftentimes people turn to self-awareness as a "quick fix" instead of putting in the necessary work to become mindfulness as a whole. We think that simply noticing something within' ourselves is enough, and giving adequate attention to that part of ourselves is not necessary.

It is not enough, however, to simply become self-aware. Doing this may allow you to know yourself more, but it will not allow you to take total control over your mind and shape it in the way that you desire. Mindfulness allows you to purposefully act with intention and objectively make decisions. Instead of being self-aware that you tend to get angry when a certain thing happens and then recognizing your angry response, you will recognize that anger and then start to understand the trigger. You will then learn to heal that trigger within' yourself and as a result you will be able to look at the trigger objectively in the future. Instead of reacting with an emotionally charged reaction, you will respond with an objectively considered response.

Mindfulness means that you will be operating in a way that will likely remove the instant gratification from most things that you do in your life. However, it will encourage a long-term sustainable state of peace that will bring you more in the long run. Instead of chasing fleeting moments of gratification and experiencing periods of suffering in between, you will teach yourself to live in a permanent state of peace that will eventually become void of those intermittent periods of suffering. As a result, your life overall will be more fulfilling with peace and in many cases, happiness.

As you read about mindfulness, especially based on the Buddhist and Dharma teachings, you may feel as though you need to go to the extent of becoming a monk and dedicating your entire life to mindfulness teachings. This is simply not true. You can live in a mindful state no matter who you are, no matter what religion you follow, and no matter where you are in life. There are no boundaries on who can practice mindfulness in this way.

Chapter Summary:

- No moment is more valuable than the rest, all are valuable to your growth
- Acknowledge each moment for what it truly is
- Setting intention allows you to consciously direct your mind
- Mindfulness eliminates instant gratification but introduces long-term gratification
- You do not need to be a monk to benefit from or achieve mindfulness

Part 2: The Science

Although mindfulness is often associated with spiritual practices, there is actually a lot of science behind it to back it up. In Buddhism and Dharma, the scientific and practical elements of mindfulness are emphasized and focused on throughout all of the teachings. In this book, you are going to learn all about these scientific and practical methods and how they directly relate to your life and your own state of mindfulness.

This section is going to specifically focus on the science behind mindfulness. As a result, you will learn exactly how this state of consciousness truly can transform your life.

Chapter 4: The Marks of Existence

In Buddhism, there are three marks of existence that describe the characteristics of everything within' the physical world, including mental activity and psychological experience. Most can agree that these three marks truly exist and that they can be found in virtually everything on the physical plane of existence. These three characteristics include impermanence, suffering, and egolessness or non-self. When you thoroughly examine and become aware of these marks, you will have an easier time abandoning the grasping and clinging tendencies that bind us together.

Impermanence (Anicca)

The idea of impermanence is that it is the fundamental property of everything that is conditioned. That means that everything that is conditioned is impermanent and that it is in a constant state of flux. Knowing this, everything that is in a state of flux and that is impermanent has the ability to be liberated.

Throughout our entire life, we attach ourselves to things, emotional states and ideas. Whenever something changes, dies, or cannot be replicated, we enter states of anger, envy, and sadness. Because of our tendency to see ourselves as permanent things and to see other things and people as permanent things as well, we tend to cling to them deeply. While we deeply cling to them, we fail to realize the deeper understanding that all things, even ourselves, are impermanent. They do not exist forever and therefore they cannot possibly exist within' our lives forever.

When you abandon the idea that you are permanent, you give yourself the chance to be liberated from the clinging that you experience with things that you desire, as well as the negative effects that arise when those things change around you. As a result, you give yourself the ability to release your fears, disappointments, and regrets that you experience when these natural and inevitable changes take place. You give yourself the ability to be liberated from these feelings and experiences and give yourself the chance to be as enlightened as you possibly can be.

When you are able to nourish your insight into impermanence on a daily basis, you have the ability to live a deeper existence, experience less suffering, and gain more enjoyment out of life. When you are able to live in the moment and appreciate all that is occurring around you here and now, you are able to experience deeper gratitude for it and thus will end up feeling more peaceful and oftentimes happier as well. From this state, when you encounter experiences where you feel pain and suffering, you know that it is impermanent and that it too shall pass.

The lesson of impermanence is something that is not regarded often in today's society. We have a tendency to cling desperately to the things that we desire and greatly fear any changes that take place around us. Yet, things are changing around us possibly faster than ever before. It may even be the rapid speed of change that further encourages our need to cling harder to the things we care so deeply about. If you think about it, though, this gives even more reason as to why you should be learning about the teachings of impermanence.

These days, material goods are a major part of society. We all have vast amounts of material possessions, whether we are considered wealthy or poor. You may look around you right now and realize the number of objects that lie around you. Even if you are an individual who lives a minimalist lifestyle, it is not hard for you to venture out and discover a space that is loaded with material possessions. Many times we put a great emphasis on these possessions and cling to them tightly. When one breaks or becomes misplaced, we enter a state of anger, fear, or sadness. In reality, this item likely had nothing to do with our ability to survive. Instead, it was something that we attached happiness to and that we failed to realize the impermanence of. As a result, when it was inevitably removed from our lives, we felt painful emotions.

More than just objects can invoke this feeling within' our lives, though. People, pets and even plants and other living beings all tend to carry profound meanings in our lives. We care deeply for the living beings that we surround ourselves with, and we often forget that they are impermanent as well. Just because someone comes in your life doesn't mean that they will stay. Even if they have been in your life for a lengthy amount of time, it doesn't promise that they will be there forever. Eventually the inevitable will occur and they will be removed from your existence, or you from theirs.

In Western culture, the topic of death is one that is often skirted or avoided altogether. We dislike the idea of impermanence so much that our entire culture avoids it and its meaning. We prefer to ignore the inevitable fate of death. Then, when it inevitably arises, we become profoundly pained, angered and saddened by its occurrence. Due to our fear of impermanence, we suffer even worse when we lose those that we care about. While that is not to suggest that mindfulness will completely change your experience and eliminate the grieving period, it does mean that being mindful will enable you to more thoroughly enjoy your time with said beings and feel deeper gratitude for their company. Then, when the inevitable does happen, you will be able to grieve knowing what you've always known: one way or another, it would end this way. Whether you lost them to death or to a change in life plans and paths, you will grieve, but you will be accepting of this inevitable loss. It will be easier for you to endure than one who never considered it or gave thought to the inevitable experience of loss due to the natural law of impermanence.

"You can't stop the waves, but you can learn to surf."

– *Jon Kabat-Zinn*

Just as Jon Kabat-Zinn says in the above quote, there truly is no way to stop the inevitable laws of life. Impermanence is one of those laws, and there is nothing that anyone can do to change that or buy extra time. As previously mentioned, we only get so many trips around the sun before our time to move on comes. The best thing you can do is to recognize this and embrace each moment with those people and things that you cherish and love most. This includes yourself, as one day you, too, will pass on. Neither you nor anyone or anything else on this entire planet is permanent. Even the earth itself will one day pass on, making way for new life or existence in the universe.

By learning to ride the waves of life and surf them, you give yourself the best chance to mindfully experience each present moment and gain the most from it that you can. You give yourself the ability to live from a peaceful state of existence and distinguish the possibility for excessive disappointment, grief, anger or sadness that arrives when impermanence proves its truth and takes away what cannot possibly last forever.

Suffering (Dukkha)

The next inevitable mark of existence is suffering and is like impermanence. The word "Dukkha" loosely translates to suffering, but more directly translates to "unsatisfactory" or "imperfect". It is important to realize that suffering exists in everything and everyone.

We are all here to experience a degree of suffering on one level or another. Everything that is material and mental with a beginning and an ending and that is composed of the five skandhas (form, sensation, perception, mental formations, and consciousness) and which has not been liberated to Nirvana will be considered Dukkha or suffering. Therefore, even things that are beautiful and elegant and pleasant experiences themselves are dukkha.

Through the Buddha's teachings, we learn that there are three primary states of suffering. The first state of suffering is pain itself, and is translated from dukkha-dukkha. This state of suffering encompasses physical, emotional and mental pains. The next type of suffering is suffering relating to impermanence or change. This suffering is translated to "viparinama-dukkha". This means that everything that you experience will soon be gone, including happiness. Because of this, you should emphasize your opportunity to enjoy it while it is existing, and prevent yourself from clinging to it so that you don't experience unnecessary pain or suffering when it disappears. The third and final state of suffering relates to conditioned states. This is translated to "samkhara-dukkha" and means that we are affected by and dependent on other things. Because of this dependency and these experiences, we are directly affected by them and this causes states of suffering within' us.

Non-Self or Egolessness (Anatta)

The third and final mark of existence is inevitable, as all three marks are. This state is called the non-self or egolessness, and is translated to Anatta, or "anatman" in Sanskrit. This teaching helps you learn that you are not a whole or independent entity. Rather, the ego or the individual self is actually considered to be a by-product of the five skandhas, which you may remember are form, sensation, perception, mental formations, and consciousness.

The five skandhas give us the illusion that we are a self and that we are individual and separate from all other living beings in this universe. But, just as everything in life, the five skandhas are consistently undergoing change and are also subject to impermanence. The not-so-simple truth is that you are not the same for two consecutive moments. Realizing this can be a difficult journey that takes a long time, and in some traditions, it is believed that this is only possible by monks. In life, we naturally cling to who we think we are, and we fail to realize that we are never the same from moment to moment. Just as everything else, we ourselves are impermanent. More so than just the fact that we eventually will die. But also because we change so frequently that we are never the same person for too long in our life.

These three marks of existence are ones that are inevitable in life. There is no possibility for you to eliminate them completely from your life, as they are a fundamental part of life itself. All of the experiences you have in life contribute to one or more of these marks of existence in one way or another. Still, the practice of becoming mindful gives you the opportunity to become deeply aware of these and act with a deeper level of understanding in mind. Instead of living at the mercy of these three marks, you can take them into consideration with your conscious decisions and use them as a guiding factor when you are making decisions in your life. These three marks of existence give you a deeper sense of what your unenlightened experience is, and give you the opportunity to shape your mindset and your life as a result.

Chapter Summary:

- The three marks of existence are present in everyone's life
- The three marks include: Impermanence (Anicca), suffering (dukkha), and not-self or egolessness (Anatta)
- Impermanence teaches that nothing - not even ourselves - are permanent
- Suffering teaches that all life is associated with suffering
- Not-self teaches that we are not whole beings all on our own

Chapter 5: Four Noble Truths

The journey of mindfulness through the teachings of Buddha and Dharma include the recognition of the four noble truths. These four noble truths are the four central beliefs that contain the essence of the entire Buddhist teachings. You will now learn what these four noble truths are, and how they directly relate to your journey to mindfulness. Remember, this journey and these truths are open to anyone who desires to lead a more mindful and peaceful existence. You are not required to be a part of any specific religion or to be a monk to learn about and grow from these beliefs. They are simply teachings that are open to anyone who desires to take the inner journey to mindfulness.

Noble Truth #1: Suffering Exists

The Buddhist view is that all life consists of varying levels of suffering and dissatisfaction. As you have already learned, this type of suffering is called Dukkha.

The very nature of humanity is imperfect, and so is the world in which you live. Throughout your entire lifetime, you will inevitably endure various degrees of physical suffering. This includes pain, injury, sickness, old age, tiredness, and eventually death. This type of suffering is especially true for people who are poor.

Knowing this, you can realize that you are never able to permanently keep all that you strive for, and that eventually, everything will pass you by. Happiness will pass you by, and eventually, you yourself will pass by, too.

Noble Truth #2: Suffering Arises from Attachment to Desires

We all inevitably suffer, just as we all inevitably have desires. The specific desires that are considered in this teaching are those relating to the desire to control things, such as cravings and sensual pleasures. This type of suffering is called "samudaya" or "tanha". An example of this type of suffering is if you desire for fame and fortune. As a result of your desires, you are destined to experience the suffering that comes with disappointment and in that path, you may even cause suffering to others around you.

When you attach yourself or your emotions to material things, you create suffering within' yourself because attachments don't last, and due to the law of impermanence, loss is inevitable. As a result of these

33

experiences, attachment to desires leads to the necessary following of suffering.

Noble Truth #3: Suffering Ceases when Attachment to Desire Ceases

Naturally, if you are able to cease your attachment to material things, then you cease the suffering that comes with that attachment. The ending of suffering in this way is called "nirodha". This means that you have successfully achieved Nirvana, which is the state you enter when you finally liberate yourself from suffering. When you enter Nirvana, your mind experiences complete liberation, freedom, and non-attachment. In this state, you are able to let go of any desire or craving. Nirvana is the process of attaining the state of dispassion.

When you achieve Nirvana, you achieve a state where you are free from all worries, all troubles, and all ideas. As much as you may try, it is impossible to comprehend this state unless you, yourself, achieve it.

Noble Truth #4: Freedom from Suffering is Possible by Practicing the Eightfold Path

The path to end suffering is known as the "Eightfold Path". This path allows you to attain liberation from suffering and is often what is referred to as "enlightenment" by many people.

The path that enables you to end suffering in your life is gradual and occurs as you continue on the journey of self-improvement through eight elements. Believe it or not, the Eightfold Path can actually extend over many lifetimes, throughout which every individual rebirth you experience is subject to karmic conditioning. Through each lifetime you will notice that the sufferings associated with cravings, ignorance, and other effects will gradually disappear. When they have completely disappeared, then you have achieved the state of Nirvana.

The Eightfold Path

As you realize that the Eightfold Path is the path to liberation from suffering, you may wish to learn more about what this path is. This path is one that you must take if you desire to totally free yourself from suffering.

The following eight attitudes or paths are the "right" or correct things that you must do in life:

1. Right View
2. Right Intention
3. Right Speech
4. Right Action
5. Right Livelihood
6. Right Effort
7. Right Mindfulness
8. Right Concentration

When you achieve this "right" way of life, you can successfully achieve Nirvana. As you can see, mindfulness itself is one of the noble truths, and as you read this book you will learn exactly how you can achieve the Right Mindfulness along your journey.

As you read about the Buddhist terms of suffering, you should realize that it is not the same as the English definition of suffering. In English, suffering implies that a person is in dire need of something in order to survive. In Buddhist teachings, suffering implies that we are all in a constant state of suffering, which we are not.

In understanding the four noble truths and the marks of existence, you can come to realize some profound things about your success in life. Due to the inevitable existence of impermanence, you can assure that you will never be living in the same situation for too long. For some period of time, you may find that you are struggling deeply and that it feels as though hard times are persistent. However, knowing the law of impermanence means that you can feel confident that very soon you will be enduring good times once again. Likewise, you must realize that good times are also impermanent and life can turn around in an instant and the troublesome times will arise once again.

It is best for your success if you do not remain attached to specific outcomes or situations. You should not become attached to actually achieving success, because then when it disappears inevitably, you will suffer more than you may have if you recognized that it would soon be gone. Still, knowing that success will come and go just like the bad times will come and go, it doesn't mean you should not maintain goals in your life. Having a positive purpose and working towards positive goals allows you to have a more peaceful and happy life overall, which is important. Those who do not have goals to work towards will end up having more hard times than positive, which leads to a lack of balance and a lack of internal peace.

"We are shaped by our thoughts; we become what we think.
When the mind is pure, joy follows like a shadow that never leaves".

– Buddha

As Buddha himself says, you need to recognize the importance of your thoughts, and therefore keeping them positive and maintaining your mindfulness no matter what situation you are in. Doing so will allow you to carry a mind that is pure, and therefore you will be able to lead a life filled with joy and happiness. It is important that you always maintain a clear awareness of your thoughts and stay mindful of what you allow to come in and how you allow it to affect you. As a result, you will be able to lead a life rich with inner peace.

Chapter Summary:

- There are four noble truths in life
- They are: suffering exists, suffering arises from attachment to desires, suffering ceases when attachment to desires ceases, freedom from suffering is possible by the eightfold path
- The eightfold path includes eight "rules" of life that can assist you in reaching nirvana
- You should still maintain a positive mind despite being in hard times and knowing hard times will come back.
- We become what we think

Chapter 6: The Three Poisons

In life, there are three poisons that can lead you towards carrying an enormous amount of emotional baggage. These poisons are ones that are easy to become entangled in, especially if you are not mindful of your thoughts. They are persistent, and once you allow yourself to fall into the pattern of one, the other two will inevitably surface. You will be lead down a path of continuously growing emotional baggage until you become aware of this cycle and develop mindfulness around it. Only then will you be able to relieve yourself from these three poisons and return to a pure mind and heart.

The Three Poisons are the cause of all human suffering, according to Buddhism. They include greed, anger, and ignorance. Whenever you read or hear about these traits, they are called the fundamental evils or the Three Poisons. These are dangerous toxins that exist in life and we must learn to eliminate them if we desire to carry on down the path to Nirvana. Under each of the Three Poisons are additional branches of said poison that can further damage your purity and carry you deeper into the toxicity of their existence.

Anger

The first of the Three Poisons is anger. This poison is accompanied by hatred, aversion, and animosity. When you are affected by greed, you may notice you are experiencing symptoms of the previous three emotions, as well as hostility, dislike, or ill-will when you are wishing harm of any sort upon another person. When you are experiencing this poison, you may find that you are resisting against many things. You will be in denial and likely will avoid any feelings that are unpleasant to you. The things you avoid may include people, places, things or specific situations. When you are being affected by this poison, you wish for everything to be satisfying all of the time. You crave and desire only comfort and pleasantness. When you are infected with this toxin, you will find that you only seem to discover more anger and hatred in your life. You are likely never calm, as you are always feeling as though you need to protect yourself from others. You fail to be able to clearly understand life for what it is and carry negative and pessimistic judgments against everything that occurs. You will likely also be creating a significant amount of your own discomfort and conflict within' yourself as a result of having an aversion to all that makes you feel uncomfortable and therefore resisting things that are important to your growth and well-being. When you are infected with the poison of hatred, you will find that you are consistently creating conflict and that you seem to have a number of enemies around you and within' you.

Greed

The second of the Three Poisons is greed. When you are greedy, you have what they call an "unquenchable third" (tahna) or intense craving for the objects you desire. You feel as though the objects you desire or the situation you desire will bring you long and lasting fulfillment, that it will make you feel whole or somehow complete. As a result, you develop a hunger for possessions or situations that ends with you striving for a goal that you will never attain because you will always set the bar higher and higher. When you are intoxicated with the poison of greed, you believe that your happiness is dependent upon you reaching a goal, and you will constantly look outside of you for things that can only be developed within' you. Greed is the never ending chase for instant gratifications that provide you with fleeting insights of the feelings you crave: happiness, joy, fulfillment, and peace. Eventually, though, greed leads to emptiness. Even the situations that once gave you fleeting happiness will eventually cease to bring you anything, and you will continually chase a feeling that is no longer available to be acquired from outside of you. You will be forced to turn inward to discover them again, should you decide to lead a life with these fundamental things we all truly want.

When you experience symptoms of greed, you will be compulsive, destructive, and impulsive. You will constantly want more and you will make instantaneous decisions with the intention to bring yourself more. You will not be thinking for your highest good, nor will you be thinking for the collective good of humankind. When you are affected by greed, it affects you on a number of different levels. It affects your success, your personal life, and your inner life. We can see the effects of greed on the globe through warfare and global conflict, which are obvious symptoms of the corporate and political greed within' our Earth. It is important that we do not fall into the path of greed, and that if we do we become mindful of our situation and break it immediately. Doing this will eliminate this poison from you and take away the suffering that is attached with greed. You will then be able to work towards a purer mind, heart, body and soul.

Ignorance

The final and possibly worst of the Three Poisons is ignorance or delusion. When we fall into a pattern of ignorance, we fall into one of the most toxic of all of the poisons. Ignorance leads to further anger and greed, which can lead to further ignorance, and take you deep into a spiral of unwanted toxicity and poison. When you are in a state of ignorance, you will be carrying a misperception of reality and the way the world works. You will fail to understand the way things actually are, and you will be influenced by your ignorance. In this state, you lack harmony with yourself, others, and the world around you. You are not able to understand the way life is interdependent and lacks permanence, therefore you will constantly look outside of yourself for happiness (greed). As you find that you are not able to discover that which you desire most, you will become frustrated and full of hatred (anger). Ignorance is the final state where you slide on the downward spiral of increasing greed and anger, and thus increasing ignorance.

When you reach the state of ignorance, you self-manifest infinitely more greed and anger into your life on an even faster level than you would if you were void of ignorance. As a result, you will find that you are constantly attracting more and more negativity to yourself, and you will not have an easy time eliminating this emotional baggage from your mind. You will be deeply affected by the Three Poisons, and it will take a large situation to eliminate these from your life. Until you can become awakened to your ignorance, you will never be able to free yourself from the Three Poisons.

The root to all emotional baggage in life is the Three Poisons. When you are infected by either of the three or any combination, you will be left with a large amount of emotional baggage that weighs heavy in your life. You will struggle to find peace and purity in your life and as a result, you will feel heavy and ill at all times. You will fail to be at harmony with yourself and the life that surrounds you, and you will have no hope of achieving nirvana.

If you recognize any of these Three Poisons in your life, it is important that you start becoming mindful around them and that you start eliminating them from your life. Eliminating them does not mean that you will not feel anger, greed, or ignorance in your life. It means that you will become aware of the situations that trigger those feelings and you will be able to act intentionally and purposefully to prevent yourself from feeding into either of them and increasing their negative impact on your life. Instead of being owned by your feelings, you will own your feelings and you will be able to powerfully control them and thus eliminate any major impact that they may have on you should you fail to recognize them.

Chapter Summary:

- There are Three Poisons in life
- The Three Poisons are anger, greed, and ignorance
- You can be infected by one, two, or all three of these poisons
- They prevent you from achieving purity or nirvana
- Ignorance is the worst, as it magnifies anger and greed

Chapter 7: Karma and Vipaka

A common "law" of life which you may be aware of is karma. Karma means what you sow you shall reap, or what you put into the world will always come back to you. On the other hand, there is vipaka, which is essentially the maturation of karma: it is when karma comes back to serve you what you have handed out. These are two very important things to consider in life, especially as you are journeying into a mindful existence.

When you are thinking about karma, you should understand that it is a basic law of life. When you put something out into the world, it is inevitable that you will get it back in some way, shape or form. For example, if you wish ill health on someone else, it is inevitable that yourself or someone you care deeply about will be affected by ill health. When that ill health comes to fruition in your own life, you will be facing vipaka. In other words, you will be facing the reality of the karma you have earned for yourself.

Karma and vipaka are not cause-and-effect in the sense of physical reactions and situations. If you rip the top off of a plant and it dies, that is not karma and vipaka. Karma and vipaka are pertaining to what you experience in your mind and the direct reactions or consequences of your actions in life based on how they affect you personally. Karma is something you cannot avoid, and you cannot escape. You *will* face the vipaka of your karma one day, one way or another.

In Buddhism, there is a common lesson taught around karma that makes it easier to understand. This lesson makes it easy for you to see why karma is important and how vipaka plays into it. When you understand the karma of your actions and learn that karma is inevitable, it makes it easier to become more mindful over what you are doing in your life.

"When a bird is alive, it eats ants. When the bird dies, ants eat the bird. Time and circumstances can change at any time. Don't devalue or hurt anyone in life. You may be powerful today. But, remember, time is more powerful than you are! One tree makes a million match sticks, but it only takes one matchstick to burn a million trees. So, be good and do good."

–   Buddha

This is a powerful quote that can really lead you to think about how life works. Karma is inevitable and it comes from every single action you take in life. Knowing that, karma can be positive or it can be negative. You can infuse the world with your positivity and have positive karma as a result and therefore positive vipaka will inevitably come to fruition in the future. Or, you can infuse the world with negativity and carry negative karma as a result, which means that when your karma ripens and vipaka happens, you will have negative situations come into fruition. One reality that you should consider is that there will always be both karmas present in your life. You will never be able to fully distinguish the negative karma. However, you can become mindful over how you view the vipaka of the karma and what response you choose as a result.

When you manage to understand karma and use it to your advantage, you can start learning how to increase the positive energy flow in your life. Although you cannot dissolve the negative, you can reduce how much it affects you and therefore have a more positive outcome in the long run. Additionally, you can recognize negative vipaka and use it to create positive karma in the future so long as you are truly mindful and intentional about how you respond to the situation.

What Causes Karma?

The primary cause of karma is ignorance. When you are unaware of how things truly are, you tend to create circumstances that warrant karma. Greed and craving what you desire is another situation that can cause karma, as there are many individuals who will do ill-willed things to fulfill their greedy cravings. In karma, the door is volition, which essentially means will. When you willfully do something without considering the outcomes, you run the chance of having greater karma. Alternatively, there is feeling which represents the vipaka. This is when you feel the result of your karma as it plays out full circle.

Are There Different Types of Karma?

You may be surprised to note that there are many types of karma that you may carry with you in life. These karmas each have their own cause and often their own outcome. They are ones that can be harvested for many years or ones that can be easily let go of. That itself is largely based off of the person who is carrying the karma and what they to in order to deal with said karma. The different types of karma are reproductive karma, supportive karma, obstructive or counteractive karma, destructive karma, weighty karma, proximate or death-proximate karma, habitual karma, and reserve or cumulative karma. Additionally, there are immediately effective karma, subsequently effective karma, indefinitely effective karma, and defunct or ineffective karma. All of these different types of karma are important to understand as each can affect you in a different way.

Reproductive Karma

Believe it or not, every single birth of a being into this world is affected by karma. The karma you carry at birth is based on the karma that was never brought to maturity at death in your past life. Therefore, you will be carrying that karma with you in your current life, good or bad. When you die, it is considered to be only a temporary end for a temporary phenomenon in the Buddhist teachings. Buddhists believe in reincarnation, meaning that you can carry karma with you for several lifetimes before it finally reaches maturity and comes to fruition. As a result, you can end up experiencing things that may seem "unfair" to you in this lifetime, because you are carrying that from a past life experience. The last thought you have in your past life before death is the thought that will determine the state you are in when you are birthed into your next life.

Supportive Karma

This type of karma is one that supports the reproductive karma. It is neither bad nor good in nature, and it is persistent through your entire lifetime. From the moment you are conceived until the moment you die, you will have supportive karma in your life. If you have moral supportive karma, you will be assisted in good health, wealth, happiness and everything else that will fulfill and enrich your life and assist in bringing you joy and contentment. However, if you have immoral supportive karma, you will be assisted in receiving pain, sorrow, misery and more. The supportive karma which you carry is one that you carry based off of what your reproductive karma is. Therefore, if you carry a positive reproductive karma, you will carry a moral supportive karma. However, if you carry a negative reproductive karma, you will then carry an immoral supportive karma.

Obstructive or Counteractive Karma

This karma tends to weaken, interrupt and disassemble the fruition of reproductive karma. For example, let's say you were born with good reproductive karma, you may be subject to experiencing various ailments and such that would prevent you from enjoying all of the wonderful results of your great actions in this lifetime. Alternatively, if you were someone who was born with bad reproductive karma and yet you lead a life full of wealth, joy, and peace, despite your negative actions in your lifetime, then that would also be the presence of obstructive or counteractive karma. This type of karma can completely switch what outcome you have from the karma in your lifetime.

Destructive Karma

The law of karma states that the powerful energy associated with reproductive karma may be eliminated if there were a powerful opposing karma from the past. This karma may be seeking the opportunity to operate and therefore finds it's window of opportunity and comes to fruition. As a result, it can not only obstruct but completely destroy the entire force of the existing karma. When you experience destructive karma, it could present as either a bad karma or a good karma.

An example of destructive karma would be if you were someone with good reproductive karma leading a good life with moral supportive karma and you then decided to kill someone out of greed or anger. As a result, you could be faced with destructive karma that would completely destroy your good karma and turn everything around for you, not only in this lifetime but potentially in many subsequent lifetimes as well. Alternatively, if you were someone with inherently bad karma and immoral supportive karma but you did something extremely positive and good, you could wind up experience destructive karma in a sense that it obstructs and destroys all of your negative karma and turns you around to have only good karma and moral supportive karma from that point on. You may continue experiencing this good karma for many lifetimes to come, as well.

Weighty Karma

When you are carrying weighty karma, it is serious. As with the previous karmas, it can be either good or bad. This karma produces results quickly, either in this life or in the next life. If you were to carry good weighty karma, for example, you would likely experience ecstasy and joy in your life as a result. Alternatively, if you were to experience immoral weighty karma, you would quickly be faced with unwanted and negative consequences that you would have to pay as a result of your actions.

Proximate or Death-Proximate Karma

This is the dying-thought-karma. It is the one that sets the tone for your reproductive karma. Proximate or death-proximate karma relates to what you do or remember immediately before you die. This karma has a powerful ability to contribute to what you will experience in your next life, and as a result, there are many traditions around this in Buddhist countries. In these countries, they often remind dying individuals of the good deeds they have done and encouraging them to do good acts on their death bed to ensure that they are blessed with the good reproductive karma in their next life.

Knowing this, a bad person has the ability to die with happy final thoughts and therefore be born with good reproductive karma. Alternatively, a good person may die unhappily or with a sudden final memory of something evil they have done in the past, and therefore they will be born with bad reproductive karma in the next life. It is important to understand this type of karma and therefore become mindful of your thoughts, then, to ensure a good reproductive karma and moral supportive karma in your next life.

Habitual Karma

When you experience habitual karma, you are experiencing karma for the things you do without recognizing you are doing it. Habits are often second nature to people, and frequently become a part of their character as a person. If one is not being mindful, they may find that they fall into their habitual mindset, which can lead to ignorance. Habitual karma is something you experience when you fall into habit and do something that is normal for you at the right or wrong time, essentially.

Reserve or Cumulative Karma

All actions that do not fall into any of the previously discussed karma bodies are ones that fall into reserve or cumulative karma. These are essentially a reserve fund or savings account of karma for a particular being. As with other karmas, they will inevitably be dealt in one lifetime or another. Just like with previous karmas, this one has the ability to be affected by obstructive or destructive karma, and thus an individual may not experience the outcome of their karmic reserves.

Immediately Effective Karma

When you experience immediately effective karma, it means that you experience the karmic outcome in this lifetime. Immediately effective karma may be experienced, for example, if you were to wish ill-health on someone you did not like and then you yourself contracted ill health in this lifetime. You may even contract the exact type of ill-health or ill-will that you wished upon someone else.

Subsequently Effective Karma

When you experience something in your next life, this is called subsequent karma. It is karma that you earn in this life that you experience in the next life. An example may be if you were to do something extremely kind for someone, and then as a result in your next life when you had a dire need for it, someone did something extremely kind for you.

Indefinitely Effective Karma

There is another type of karma called indefinite karma, which can also be known as defunct or ineffective karma. This karma does not take place in the next life, but rather it takes place at any time in your lifetimes until you attain nirvana.

Defunct or Ineffective Karma

When karma does not operate in this life at all, it is called defunct or ineffective karma. This means that it did not serve you in this life to teach you a lesson and therefore it becomes ineffective. You may not know in your next life what it was that caused said karma, so it loses its impact.

Understanding the many varieties of karma can allow you to understand why certain things may occur in your life and become mindful over their existence. You can begin to recognize areas of your life where ignorance may be taking place and replace that ignorance with awareness and mindfulness, and thus reduce or eliminate your karma. As well, you should understand the importance of death-proximity karma and reproductive karma. These are ones that have a profound impact on your lifetime of karma. Finally, understanding obstructive and destructive karmas are important, too, as they can completely change the way your karma is judged.

Vipaka is the process by which karma comes to maturity and is experienced. It is directly related to karma and is present in every form of karma. When you experience karma, which is inevitable, you will experience vipaka, which is also inevitable. You may experience the vipaka in this lifetime, or you may experience it in a later lifetime if it is defunct or ineffective karma. One way or another, though, you will experience it.

Chapter Summary:

- Karma is a moral law of cause and effect
- Vipaka is the term for when karma matures and the effect is experienced
- There are many different types of karmas which you can be affected by
- You may experience karma from a past life
- Buddhists believe you can control your karma for your next life based on your dying thoughts

Chapter 8: Five Precepts

There are five precepts pertaining to Buddhist teachings that are essentially immoral actions that one should refrain from in their lifetime. Taking part in this five precepts leads to emotional baggage, karma, and an inability to achieve nirvana. In addition to the five precepts that are important for everyone, there are five more that pertain to Buddhist monks. Of course, you do not need to worry about the ones associated with Buddhist monks, but for informative and educational purposes we will discuss those as well.

The Five Precepts

The five precepts are simple to understand and follow and they make complete sense as to why they exist. These precepts are ones that Buddhists believe that all people should refrain from, should they desire to live a life free of emotional baggage. When you partake in these precepts, you expose yourself to the development of excessive emotional baggage that can lead to unhappiness, ill-health, and an otherwise negative or unfulfilling life. The five precepts are:

- Harming living things
- Taking what is not given
- Sexual misconduct
- Lying or gossiping
- Taking intoxicating substances such as alcohol or drugs

These five precepts are basically the five laws of "what not to do" that Buddhists live by. In doing so, it saves them from an enormous amount of emotional baggage that they may otherwise carry if they were to engage in these activities. When you engage in any of these five precepts, you will end up carrying experiences of misery, guilt, sadness, anger, greed, and ignorance. As you can see, the results of these five precepts contains all of the Three Poisons which Buddhists look to avoid. In mindfulness practice, it makes sense that you too would want to avoid the Three Poisons and therefore activities that would cause them. In addition to the emotional baggage that these experiences bring about, you would also expose yourself to bad karma, potentially even destructive karma that could destroy your good karma and leave you with a lifetime of bad karma.

The Five Additional Precepts for Monks

While you are not expected to become a monk, nor do you need to be in order to have a strong mindfulness practice, it is always interesting to further explore the teachings that you are learning about. In Buddhist traditions, monks have five additional precepts that they must follow, meaning that they have ten in total. Their additional precepts are:

- Eating substantial amounts of food in midday (from noon to dawn)
- Dancing, singing, or listening to music
- Using garlands, perfumes and personal adornments such as jewelry
- Using any sort of luxurious bed or seating
- Accepting or holding money, silver or gold

The five additional precepts for Buddhist monks seem a bit extreme for those living in modern day society, particularly in the Western world; however, it is interesting to learn about. When looking at these precepts on a deeper level, they essentially assist the monk in refraining from experiencing greed, anger, or ignorance. They are taught to develop an inner sense of peace, joy, and fulfillment and to maintain it and sustain it in a more powerful way than we may understand. Again, you do not need to partake in any of these five precepts for any reason, nor do you need to become a monk in order to use the powerful teachings within' this book. This added section is merely for your entertainment and understandings! If you are looking to develop a more mindful life, you may wish to consider the reasons why Buddhists monks refrain from these five additional precepts and what these bring about in your life. Are there luxurious things that you enjoy, such as your bed or jewelry, that you may no longer notice anymore due to habitual use?

If You Engage in One of the Five Precepts

The five precepts are essentially a guide in teaching you to live an ethical life. At the very least you should apply these five precepts in order to ensure that you are living life ethically and without the intention of doing harm or ill-will to yourself or anyone else in this lifetime or any other lifetime. If you were to engage in one of the five precepts, you would experience an incredible amount of emotional baggage and karmic build up as a result. Crossing the five precepts would lead you into unethical or immoral territory, which would naturally lead you into immoral karma. You would inevitably experience bad vipaka as a result. In addition to your bad vipaka, you would also experience emotional baggage that would lead you away from nirvana. You would then need to put forth all of the extra mindfulness work to retrace your steps and lead you back into a path of purity and peace to restore all that you lost when you crossed the ethical ways of life.

The five precepts are set up to help you lead an ethical life that will assist you in carrying good karma and a pure mind, heart, body and soul. When you lead a life in alignment with the five precepts, you ensure that you are going to have a positive existence with long term gratification and fulfillment. You eliminate the emotional baggage and bad karma that arises as a result of crossing the five precepts, which is something that is commonly done in western culture. As a result, you increase your mindfulness practice and lead yourself closer to nirvana.

Chapter Summary:

- The five precepts are five ethical rules of life
- The five precepts include: do no harm, do not take what is not given, do not engage in sexual misconduct, do not lie or gossip, and do not take intoxicating substances.
- Buddhist monks have five additional precepts in their way of life
- You do not have to be a Buddhist or a monk to follow these rules and gain value from them
- These five rules have a powerful ability in reducing and eliminating emotional baggage and bad karma

Chapter 9: The Middle Way

The middle way is one of the most profound teachings in Buddhism. When you adhere to the middle way, you open yourself up to a greater ability to achieve and maintain peace in your life, as well as the ability to create a more sustainable form of gratification. Instead of responding to instant gratification, which can lead to a great deal of emotional baggage in the long run, you will learn to create and sustain moderate long-term gratification. With instant gratification, you open yourself up to the constant "rollercoaster" of ups and downs. Instead, you want to learn to create a type of gratification that allows you to consistently feel good, rather than occasionally feel great.

The middle path is one which allows you to powerfully focus on the intention behind your actions and thus create a greater sense of peace overall. Instead of disregarding your intent and winding up with a negative outcome, such as stress or frustration, you can maintain your focus and thus maintain your peace. This path is not one that you should follow out of fear of being harmed by any sort of supernatural agency. Instead, it is one that you follow for the value it offers on your inner journey and for the most desirable outcome: self-purification.

When you follow this path, you will not find yourself falling into any sort of external worship or prayer. Rather, you will be guided and protected, as well as living in harmony with the universal law. Living your life by the Eightfold Path guides you directly to inner peace and purification. You can follow it much like a road map. When you do, you will learn how you can achieve Nirvana in your life.

It is important to realize that, just like a road trip with a road map, the map to Nirvana is a slower and steadier one. You must have a great deal of intention and mindfulness in order to achieve in, and thus the slower and more steady you travel, the easier and quicker you will arrive at Nirvana. If you force it or attempt to speed down the path, you are likely to end up driving yourself further away from the success of your trip.

There are three legs of your road trip: morality (known as "Sila"), mental culture (known as "Samadhi"), and wisdom (known as "Panna"). In order to achieve Nirvana from the Eightfold Path, you must develop each of these legs simultaneously, with an intensity that is appropriate to your own abilities and needs. First, you must develop your morality. Your actions need to bring good to the lives of other beings all over the globe, including yourself. You can do so by faithfully adhering to the five precepts. At the time that you start to develop morality, you will find it easier to develop the powers of concentration and thus your mental culture will develop. Finally, when your concentration develops, your wisdom will come to life and you will have accomplished your need to achieve the three legs of the journey.

You may be confused as to why there are only three legs on the journey despite there being eight "rules" on the Eightfold Path. Reasonably so. The answer is simple: the first leg, morality, covers three rules from the Eightfold Path. That is, right speech, right action, and right livelihood. Then the next leg, mental culture, covers right effort, right mindfulness, and right concentration. Finally, the leg of wisdom covers the last two rules from the Eightfold Path: right understanding and right thoughts.

It is important to understand that you will not be able to achieve all of these ways at once, nor will you be able to achieve them quickly. Each human on their own path will have a different rate at which each of these legs develops for them. It will be largely based on the intention of said person, their devotion to their personal development, and what they wish to accomplish. One who is more devoted to their inner development will have an easier journey than one who hardly cares about their development at all.

It is vital that you have a strong intention behind your actions and your desire to grow. The more intention you hold for your development, the easier you will be able to accomplish anything you set your mind to. The intention of your actions, thoughts, and desires are extremely powerful and important.

Once you have a strong understanding of how the Eightfold Path works, you will be able to deeper understand the Middle Way. The Eightfold Path is powerful for helping you develop your mindfulness practice, while the Middle Way is a powerful way to help you develop your sustainable gratification. The Middle Way is simple and holds virtually one rule to it: never lack and never have too much. Always find yourself in the middle.

Let's assume you are craving something delicious to eat for supper. You know exactly what you want, and you are prepared to go out and get it. In modern society, it is not uncommon to rush to gather your things, leave the house and pick up your dinner, then rush home and rush through the meal. As a result, you hardly satisfy your craving and you certainly don't satisfy the mental aspect of it. You may even find yourself craving said food several times over until you finally feel as though you have fulfilled the craving. Additionally, as a result of your rushing, you may find yourself feeling stressed out and frustrated. Simple things may become a trigger for you to feel even more stressed out and frustrated. Your entire experience of attempting to fulfill a craving has been an unenjoyable event that even brought about negative emotions to your day. Ultimately, you have failed to create any level of gratification because you sought to fulfill your craving through instant gratification.

If, instead, you were to take things slower you would fulfill your gratification needs that night and you would do so happily. You would take your time gathering your things and getting ready. The smaller things wouldn't bug you. You would no longer feel stressed out by drivers doing the speed limit because you, too, would be doing the speed limit. Instead of risking accidents or unwanted situations, you would be able to mindfully maintain your awareness and ensure that you are keeping yourself and others on the road safe. When you arrived at the restaurant, you would take in the experience and fulfill all of your senses with it. You may even choose to sit down and eat instead of taking your food home. Or, you would take your food home but you would do so at a medium pace. When you arrived at the point of eating your food, you would sit down and ensure you were completely comfortable. You would then eat your food slowly and enjoy each bite as if it were your first. When it came to the last bite, you would feel satisfied and your craving would be fulfilled.

The Middle Way teaches us to slow down and take things in stride. It is valuable for virtually everything you do in life. When you lead your life according to the Middle Way, it does not intend for you to be to one extreme or the other. For example, one of the five precepts is not to kill. However, the Buddha himself was not a vegetarian. Instead of being extremely one way or another, it means you are slightly here and slightly there. You do not eat excessive amounts of meat, but you do not refrain from eating it at all, either. Instead, you eat what you need to derive your nutrients and that is all. It is best to ensure that you are eating all of the right items to gain total sustenance. When you turn to vegetarian supplements or other supplements to fulfill a healthful diet, you are essentially going to one extreme. You will also end up carrying unnecessary emotional baggage, such as through having to purchase extra items when you otherwise wouldn't need to.

It is important to realize that being a person on the Middle Way path does not mean that you are to never respond to anything. Let's say, for example, you were struggling with a coworker. You would not simply allow that coworker to continually bully you and treat you unkindly. Rather, you would stand up for yourself and assert your boundaries. However, you would not go further than you would need to. Instead, you would refrain from taking things to the extreme and you would assert yourself only enough to create the peace in your life that you need to, then you would move on.

The Middle Way is about refraining from taking any extreme measures in life. You should not be extremely "yes" or extremely "no". Instead, you should simply do what you need to in order to survive in a healthy and fulfilling life that is complete with sustainable gratification. Nothing more, nothing less. When you go on either end of the spectrum, either more or less, you enter into a place where you wind up having a significant amount of emotional baggage. As a result, you will suffer deeply and will end up sabotaging your ability to lead a mindful life.

You should spend time developing your ability to lead life on the Middle Way path. Doing so will increase your ability to have sustainable gratification and will eliminate the instant gratification and all of the emotional baggage that it carries alongside it in your life. When you learn to develop a sustainable level of gratification, you ensure that you will stay peaceful and pure so long as you maintain your balance and continue walking the Middle Way and don't sway to either of the extremes.

Chapter Summary:

- The Middle Way means not working on either extreme
- The Middle Way is a derivative of the Eightfold Path
- You should not be excessively giving nor excessively taking
- The Middle Way encourages you to follow the Five Precepts, too
- Leading the middle way develops balance and thus inner purity and harmony
- The Buddha himself was not a vegetarian, it is okay to get nutrition from meat. Simply don't take too much.

Chapter 10: The Five Aggregates

The Five Aggregates, also known as the Five Skandhas, are elements of our existence that work towards producing a mental being. The teaching of The Five Aggregates analyzes personal experiences and assists people in viewing cognition from Buddha's perspective. Without The Five Aggregates, a mental being would simply cease to exist. There would be no such thing. These elements are present in every living being with a mind, and therefore you can expect that just as you have them, so too does everyone else that you encounter in life.

The Five Aggregates are:

- Form
- Sensation
- Perception
- Mental Formation
- Consciousness

Aggregates are continually changing: they are not static being, rather they are dynamic. When you understand the Five Aggregates, you give yourself the opportunity to truly and purely obtain the wisdom of the not-self.

The entire world as you know it is not created upon or around the idea of self, but rather through impersonal processes. When you eliminate the idea of "self", you are able to look at happiness, suffering, praise, blame and other emotions with equality. You no longer subject yourself to imbalance because you give yourself the ability to open up and see the purpose and importance of each. You eliminate the continuous imbalances of alternating hope and fear by creating a sustainable sense of inner purity and appreciation for each of the emotions you experience.

On a deeper level, of course, each of The Five Aggregates can be observed at a greater insight. You can further understand what each of these is. These Aggregates are present and important in anyone's life, Buddhist or not, as they are inevitable and they exist everywhere. When you take the time to open yourself up to the wisdom of the aggregates, you give yourself the ability to truly understand your own mindfulness practices on a deeper level.

Form (Known as "Rupa")

The Aggregate called form discusses all that we know in the material and the physical world. Everything that is materialized in front of you is called form. Your body, your home, your car, your place of work, all of the things you encounter in the physical realm on a daily basis constitute for form. However, when we are discussing form from The Five Aggregates, we want to discuss specifically the form of your physical body. This includes five of your physical organs: (ear, nose, eye, body and tongue) and all of the corresponding physical objects associated with these aggregates. (Anything that can be seen, smelled, heard, tasted, or touched). It is clear that form exists, and it doesn't take magic to see it or know it. Your body is a physical, tangible form that you can intentionally feel in order to affirm its existence. So, too, can you do the same with anything that appeals to any of your five senses within' the physical realm.

Sensation (Known as Vedana)

There are three sensations or feelings associated with this aggregate that you need to know about. The three include: unpleasant, pleasant, and indifferent. Whenever you experience the sensation of an object, you will be able to identify one of these emotional tones associated with the experience. You may, for example, touch the end of a knife and associate and unpleasant emotional tone with it. Alternatively, you may touch a soft blanket with your bare skin and associated a positive tone with it. Finally, you may touch something that you touch on a daily basis and you have become accustomed to it and therefore you don't necessarily feel any emotions associated with the experience. In this case, you have attached an indifferent tone with the experience. When you are interacting with something in its form, you will have at least one of these sensations.

Perception (No Alternative Name)

Perception is the experience by which mental beings interpret things. When you use perception, you take an indefinite experience and you turn it into a definite, identifiable and recognizable experience. Through this, you create the conception of an idea about certain experiences or objects. Perceptions change from person to person, which means the same experience can have a different perceived reality among two or more beings. You are not likely to have the same experiences as anyone else in life. Perception is the aggregate you are working with specifically when you are increasing your mindfulness in life. It is essentially a practice of you changing how you perceive reality and the world around you, and even teaching you to further increase your ability to perceive things in a more realistic and beneficial method. By altering how you perceive things, you can increase your long-term sustainable gratification, fulfillment, and satisfaction within' life.

Mental Formation (No Alternative Name)

The conditioned response you have to an object or an experience is known as the aggregate called mental formation. This aggregate does not merely cover the impression that was created by previous actions, but it also covers the responses of here and now. The responses you experience in the here and now are motivated and directed through life in a particular way. The volatility of mental formation is powerful, considering it is so fluid. You will continually experience things in different ways, depending upon what your motivation and drive are at the time of the experience. Mental formation is a moral dimension, feeling or sensation is an emotional dimension, and perception is a conceptual dimension.

Consciousness (No Alternative Name)

The final of The Five Aggregates is consciousness. The presence of consciousness with the eye and formation are what make experiences for the mental being. Any sense you use is only experienced as a result of the presence of consciousness, meaning that you must have consciousness in order to have any worldly experiences. All mental beings have consciousness. In simple terms, consciousness is merely the awareness one has towards an object or a sensation they experience with the object. There are varying levels of consciousness that are important to consider when you are discussing consciousness in these terms. You can experience consciousness in the forms of:

- Ear consciousness (sound)
- Nose consciousness (smell)
- Body consciousness (touch)
- Eye consciousness (see)
- Tongue consciousness (taste)
- Mind consciousness (awareness)

The sixth sense of the mind is important to understand because it actually does carry its own impact in life. When we are discussing the consciousness of the mind, we are not considering physical objects that you can experience with your tangible senses. Rather, we are discussing unseen objects such as ideas or other mental activities that you experience on a regular basis.

The first five consciousness types are not related to each other in any way shape or form. However, they are all associated with mind consciousness as their coordinator. When each of the forms of consciousness is linked up with mind consciousness, it gives you the ability to formulate thoughts, ideas and perceptions around the experience you have with the other senses. So, if you were to touch something, your body consciousness would become aware of the touch. It would be your mind consciousness, however, that would allow you to formulate an opinion or idea based on said touch. The same goes for all of the remaining consciousness forms as well.

Mind consciousness has the ability to allow you to recognize and discriminate your experiences in three primary ways:

- Comparative Cognition: Your mind can compare objects despite one or both not being physically present. The comparisons may include: specific insights about quantity of items and quality of items, including things one may feature that the other does not.

- Physical Cognition: your mind can instantly reference a physical object that you are holding or experiencing in the present moment based on past experiences.
- Non-Cognition: Your mind can "create" false cognition in the absence of physical objects by mentally formulating something with an irrelevant experience and thus comparing it with something in the present moment.

The mind consciousness is a powerful thing you must learn to understand, as it controls the alternative five consciousness forms. It's ability to initiate the other forms of consciousness allow it to create all types of neutral, wholesome and unwholesome activities that keep your life in motion.

If you are an individual who has decided to follow the Buddhist way of life, there are two additional consciousness forms: the seventh consciousness (called "Klista-mano") and the eighth consciousness ("Alaya"). In regards to your mindfulness practice and development, however, you do not need to know too much about these two.

Chapter Summary:

- The Five Aggregates are parts of your mental being

- The Five Aggregates Include: form, sensation, perception, mental formation and consciousness.

- There are six primary levels of consciousness: one associated with each of the senses and one associated with the mind.

- If you are Buddhist, there are two additional consciousness formations.

- Understanding The Five Aggregates helps you deeper understand your perception of reality.

Part 3: The 21st Century

Understanding the teachings of Buddhism and how they can relate to your life can be difficult. Although you have been taught several real-life examples until now, you may still be curious as to how these teachings can directly relate to you. In some cases, the previous teachings may feel old or even outdated. The reality is, you need to understand these basic lessons in order to be able to have a solid foundation to build your own mindfulness practice on.

In this section, we are going to focus on scenarios that will be a closer to your own reality. You will learn exactly how you can take all that you have learned, plus more, and put it into action in your real life in the 21st century. These days, there are many things that simply did not exist when Buddha was alive, and as a result, we must adapt to his teachings and understand how we can actually work them into our modern lives.

You are going to learn about how social media, technology, modern food and diets, consumerism and more influence and affect your mindfulness practice. You will also learn how you can understand and become mindful over their specific influences and thus learn how you can make a profound and significant change. As a result, you will be able to increase your mindfulness practice within' your own life.

Until now, you learned about Buddhist teachings and how they respond to everyday life based on the most simplistic of lives. Many of the teachings are extremely important to modern lives, but several may not make any sense. Now is the time that you will learn to make sense of these teachings and understand how you can enforce them within your own modern life.

Once again, please remember that you are not expected to become a Buddhist. Rather, these teachings hold important keys, tools, and knowledge to assist you in understanding how to develop your own mindfulness practice. As a result, you will learn exactly how you can powerfully alter your life to create a happier, more joyful life filled with purpose and intention.

Chapter 11: Shiny Object Syndrome

In the 21st century, we are powerfully driven by something called "shiny object syndrome". That is, we crave instant gratification. Anything that provides us with an instant boost in dopamine and allows us to feel extremely good, we are willing to do it. That is why we have people known as "thrill seekers" and other such terms because we are seeking greater satisfaction out of life. We are searching for our purpose, looking for happiness, and trying to find meaning in everything.

In the 21st century, we are able to get things faster than ever, and we are able to create instant gratification. As you have learned previously in this book, though, instant gratification is not necessarily an ideal type of gratification. It leads to many ups and downs. In the moment, you are fulfilled. However, you will very quickly find that you are no longer satisfied and you must move on to the next thing rather quickly in order to feel that sense of gratification again. As a result, you go through a rollercoaster of emotions, which includes a lot of suffering. Eventually, you may even discover that your methods of obtaining instant gratification no longer serve you, and that you are no longer feeling that instant sense of joy and happiness when you engage in such an activity. So, you go on to the next thing. That is where we get thrill seekers who are seeking adrenaline rushes that give them an instant fix of happiness and satisfaction. Only, in this day and age those risk takers are finding that more and more they are dying from tragic accidents caused by their thrill-seeking desires. And in between their stunts, they are desperately searching for another sense of gratification as they find themselves feeling stagnant or bored once again. In other words, they suffer in between adrenaline "fixes".

Instant gratification actually opens the door for a lot more lows. Since you are so pressed to feel satisfied *right now* you may feel rushed for time. You may get frustrated at anything that slows you down, even if it's moving at a normal and average pace. For example, imagine you are wanting to purchase a new shirt for yourself. You saw it a few days before pay day and you wanted to have it. You knew there were plenty in stock, but you asked for the lady at the counter to put one on hold for you. Therefore, you know the one you want is available for you. Still, you are so excited that first thing on payday you jump in your car and take off. You speed to the mall and become deeply frustrated when you are slowed down by other drivers, even though they are going the speed limit. You stress and feel as though they are hogging the road, and so the joyful experience of getting your new shirt becomes the stressful experience of getting to the mall in all of the traffic, even though the traffic is only something you perceive. When you arrive at the mall, if you don't find the perfect parking stall up next to the door, you will likely be stressed that you have to walk so far, even though it isn't really that far, to begin with. If there is a line up at the store, you will be even more stressed. The entire process will bring about stress, even though everything you are encountering is perfectly normal situations that would have occurred no matter what you had done. There would be nothing you can do to alter the situation, and furthermore, none of it actually takes away from the fact that you are still getting the new shirt. Instead of enjoying the process and truly embracing the joy of the new shirt, you add a large amount of stress to your life and the shirt barely fulfills your need to feel that instant gratification. It is overshadowed by the stress. And if you share that stress with anyone else, such as through technology or when you get home, you further negate from that experience and take away how wonderful it was. Even your happy experiences are tarnished with negativity and stress. Instant gratification pays no one due happiness.

Imagine instead that you were to know that the shirt was on hold. You got up in the morning and still ate something for breakfast. You took your time getting your shoes on and got in your car and let it heat up properly while you picked a good playlist. On your way to the mall, you were driving at the flow of traffic so no one was in your way, and you got the perfect parking stall, even if it was at the back of the lot and you had to walk. You headed into the mall and when you reached the store you noticed a lineup, but the fact that you *knew* your shirt was there for you meant that it didn't matter because you were coming to get what you wanted. Instead of stressing, you spent that time enjoying the store and looking around at all of the other wonderful clothes, fantasizing about what they would feel like and getting an idea of what is in season now. Taking in all of the fashionable art. Then, when you got your shirt and left the mall, you would be feeling full of joy and gratification. There would be no stress associated with the situation. No negative things to recount to your friends either through technology or in person. The entire experience would bring you pure joy and satisfaction and you would feel a great deal of sustainable gratification from it. You may even feel amazing for the rest of the day, whereas if it were instant gratification, you may have only felt good for a fleeting moment.

Sustainable gratification is achieved through methods you have learned earlier in this book. The Middle Way, the Eightfold Path, and all of the other mindfulness practices that you learned are able to powerfully guide you in the direction of happiness and sustainable gratification. When you find your gratification through these methods, you feel grateful for something for much longer and, as a result, you eliminate the amounts of suffering you feel in regards to your gratification levels.

It may seem difficult to create sustainable gratification in your life, as you don't get instant results like you are likely accustomed to at this time. However, once you learn how to create this type of gratification in your life, you will learn how fulfilling it can be and it will satisfy you for a much longer time frame than instant gratification will. As a result, you will feel happier longer, and your inner peace will last much longer, as well.

Chapter Summary:

- Instant gratification is not sustainable
- Instant gratification leads to excessive emotional baggage
- When you rush, you destroy the joy from the experience
- Sustainable gratification allows you to deeply feel the joy of every experience
- Sustainable gratification takes more time to develop, but brings great happiness long term

Chapter 12: Technology

Technology and all of its various ways of being entwined in our modern lives has also carried a major impact in the way we experience gratification and how long we feel happy for. There are multiple ways that technology has even further increased our experiences of attaining instant gratification and inhibited our ability to acquire sustainable gratification. Don't be confused, technology is a wonderful development and has a very powerful and admirable use in society. It has created a number of wonderful advancements and assisted us in wonderful ways. However, our inability to learn to use it in a way that affects us positively has led to many negative outcomes.

As a society, technologies such as video games, the internet, phones, and other high-tech pieces have only been around for about thirty to forty years. As a result, we have not exactly learned how to use them with moderation in order to increase our enjoyment from the experience and decrease our negative outcomes. In more modern research findings, it is being discovered that prolonged use of high-tech devices in consecutive minutes or hours can lead to many negative side effects. We are lead to an even deeper sense of instant gratification as technology operates at much higher speeds than the human brain can. As a result, many people prefer technology over reality, which can lead to a number of issues on its own.

Negative Drawbacks of Technology

When you look at the alarmingly high numbers of people who prefer technology to reality, you discover a major flaw in our society. People prefer to communicate, spend time together, and play together through technology. The instantaneous outcome and the ability to take it anywhere with us makes it easy to prefer it. However, this leads to people struggling to become involved in real life situations. They have a difficult time communicating when face to face, or even when they are face to face over a screen such as through video chats. Additionally, they struggle to be in social settings due to social anxiety, and depression. Reality simply doesn't bring that instant gratification and people who are highly reliant on it struggle to create a sense of gratification within' their own life. The outcome is that people are more depressed because they struggle to create dopamine without instant fixes. They fail to be able to make happiness because they simply are no longer trained on how they can do so.

They may not even know what actually brings them happiness outside of the virtual world of technology.

Social Media

In addition to the struggles people face in reality, they also face these struggles online. Social anxiety has begun to transcend the physical world and has become firmly rooted in the technological world. On social media, people are posting things that they know will attract attention and are hiding parts of themselves that they fear will not. They become so fearful about the lack of attention that they try and dissolve certain fundamental and unique parts of themselves that are a large part of what makes them who they are, simply because they don't feel it will be well-received by others. The fear and anxiety that comes with these situations is massive.

As well as only posting what we think will get likes, other's do the same. This leads to false perceptions of realities and the belief that certain people are "perfect" when the truth is that no such thing exists. We are exposed to a number of things that we feel we should be doing as a society, and in most cases, it simply doesn't fit into reality. For example, you may follow a gym trainer and see that their body is perfectly curved and shaped. Their muscles are toned and they look great in anything they wear due to their attractive physique. You, on the other hand, may be a customer service representative or a banker. That means that unlike the gym trainer, you do not actually have the time nor the need to train many hours per day. However, because you see this person and you see the attention they get for their achievements, you develop the idea that you need to work out the way they do and eat the way they do. Then, you may also follow a makeup artist. Their makeup is their income, therefore, they are constantly make up extremely well when they are going to work or when they are marketing themselves online. So now you feel as though you need to work out constantly and always have your makeup done perfectly, otherwise, you will not be well-received by the world around you. This leads to an unhealthy perception of who we are supposed to be, which leads to anxiety and depression when we realize there simply aren't enough hours in the day to be this superhuman vision we have created in our minds.

Social media has created an extremely powerful tool to be seen by the masses. It is a great way to interact with others and make friends, but it is incredibly important that you learn how to properly respect social media for what it truly is. Having a healthy respect for it will assist you in pulling yourself away from the numbers game and enjoying social media for what it was meant to be: a place to be social. You eliminate the stress that comes from feeling as though you are constantly in a climb to be better, and you give yourself the ability and the permission to relax and enjoy life as you once did.

Video Games

Another way our instant gratification has been affected is through video games. Video games can now be found anywhere: on your computer, on your gaming console, on your mobile device, and in a number of other places. You can get video games on-the-go, or you can get them at home. They have even come out with virtual reality consoles that you strap to your face and feel as though you are truly inside of said reality. Video games are incredible, and they have a wonderful ability to do some profound and impactful things in our society. They have been used to train pilots and many safety officials. Using virtual stimulations has been an incredible tool for many companies and professions when teaching people how to master their profession without all of the potential risks of true hands-on training. It truly has a powerful impact on society on a professional level.

Video games even have a profound and positive impact on individuals when they are used properly and respected properly. They have the ability to give you a small "escape" from reality when you want to relax, and they give you the ability to expand your mind and imagination beyond where you may have been able to go on your own. However, when you start playing too much or too long, that is when video games can have a negative effect. Aside from the fact that some people struggle to decipher reality from virtual reality and wind up making extremely dangerous choices in public, video games instill a greater issue with instant gratification. You can do just about anything in a number of minutes or hours, oftentimes things that you would not be able to do in real life for a longer time. There is no sweat equity in video games, and therefore it is much easier to attain your desired outcome from them. In real life, you would likely have to work incredibly hard to accomplish even half of the things you could accomplish in a day of gaming, and even then you wouldn't be able to do many things because they simply don't exist in our world.

Gaming has instilled an unhealthy preference for virtual reality over real reality, and it has led to numerous ailments. The instant gratification that people acquire from video games encourages people to simply accomplish their desires in a virtual reality instead of in true reality. Unfortunately, the gratification you derive from a video game will never amount to the type of gratification you could create in real life if you were to accomplish a number of things in reality. However, avid video gamers fail to make the connection and instead they jump between various instant gratification pieces in a number of minutes and then fail to remove themselves from the virtual reality and do anything in real life to bring them gratification. Overall, they tend to be more depressed, anxious and stressed out.

Technology has a very positive and powerful use in society and that should not be discredited. There are many reasons why technology is here to stay, and so it should be. From medical advancements to safer career training, and even providing a wonderful connection for average people in an online space. Whether it be through social media or games, there are many wonderful friendships and connections that can be made online. However, if you are one who engages in online time, then you must remember the Middle Way rules. You do not need to be "against" technology in any sense, but you should refrain from being an extremist, either. Learning to find a healthy balance between both the virtual reality and true reality will help you have a strong appreciation for both and will make you a healthier individual overall.

Chapter Summary:

- Technology reinforces instant gratification
- Technology is important and useful in society and should be respected for that
- Excessive usage of technology can lead to unhealthy views of reality
- Some side effects include anxiety, stress, and depression
- The Middle Way path can help you create a healthy balance between the online and offline worlds

Chapter 13: Food and Diet

It is no secret that the basis of our diet has changed entirely since our ancestors were alive. In the time that Buddhism was established, people still regularly ate food directly from the Earth. Vegetables, fruits, nuts and other produce were freshly harvested or dried and stored for short periods of time. Meats were also fresh at the time, and only enough to consume was harvested for consumption. Their diets contained no preservatives or chemicals, and their salt intakes were not excessive with added salts due to its use as a preservative. The diet in those times was significantly different from the diets we are accustomed to in our modern lives. Back in the day, diets fueled people and kept their body and organs functioning optimally to keep them healthy and pure.

In modern times, food has lost its importance and has become another format for instant gratification. We have fast food, frozen meals, and many quick and convenient meal options that make it easy for us to eat on the go. Our diet is completely different from what it once was. We now harvest massive amounts of produce and meat and process it in ways that allow it to be stored for enormous amounts of time. Harvests are grown for quantities and not quality in many instances, and as a result, not all produce is the same with the same health benefits. Sometimes our soils are leached of all of their benefits and as a result farmers are forced to introduce chemical fertilizers and other soil enhancers in order to produce crops that meet the idealistic demands of our excessive diets.

There are three primary ways that our diet negatively affects our life in this day and age. The three ways include: lack of mindfulness around eating, decreased health standards, and increased instance of instant gratification leading to greater suffering.

Mindful Eating

As with every other area of your life, eating is an experience and it is one that should be enjoyed. If you ever look at a high-end restaurant, you will see that they emphasize on their quality and not their quantity. They are extremely clear on how much one needs to actually eat in order to feel satisfied, and therefore they don't encourage over-indulging. Instead, they encourage a fully mindful experience that truly entices all of the senses. Their meals are fragrant, full of flavor and texture, and are plated in a way that is beautiful to look at. These restaurants encourage consumers to have a mindful experience when you eat there. If you were to go to one and eat your food down quickly without taking your time to enjoy the experience, you would likely be frowned upon. You would miss the entire point of the experience and you would fail to truly gain the satisfaction of it all.

As a society, we have become accustomed to our fast and on-the-go lifestyles. Many individuals consume high quantities of fast and convenient foods that lack most of the parts of food that is to be enjoyed. They lack texture, taste, fragrant and appearance when you consume them. The convenience food industries know this, and so they use wax models of their meals to make them look enticing and then when you go and purchase said meal it actually looks terrible and tastes worse. The point is to encourage consumers to crave their food, and then come purchase it. Due to the convenience, consumers are compelled to do just that.

The convenience food industry destroys the experience of eating. We eat our meals quickly and fail to experience them because there isn't too much to experience with them, to begin with. They are often extremely large in proportion to what we actually need to eat because the industry knows how quickly we eat and therefore we often overindulge. Since these foods are highly salted, it often leads to an extremely ill feeling just minutes after you finish consuming the meal. At this point, the entire experience has been destroyed.

Mindfulness and eating are things that go hand-in-hand. When you bring the enjoyment of eating back into the picture, you will actually find that you eat healthier. Eating convenient and fast foods slowly is not as pleasurable as they lack taste and texture. In many cases, they actually taste gross. It also encourages you to eat slowly and therefore you truly feel when you are full and you stop eating, typically much sooner than you would if you were quickly indulging in a fast food meal. As a result, you end up feeling much more satisfied and you are not ill afterward. The experience is pleasurable from beginning to end.

Decreased Health Standards

The physical health deterioration caused by eating convenience foods that are highly processed is easy to see. When you look at the general public, particularly in Western culture, you can see exactly how the low food standards have completely changed the general image of society. People are experiencing more and more ailments. Not just obesity, but diabetes, cancer, anxiety, heart attacks and many other health ailments are increased by our poor diet standards. When people are ill on a physical level, they are not able to feel as in tune with their inner selves and achieve the inner purification and happiness that we all desire.

Additionally, when you can physically see how damaging the effects have been externally, you must then be able to imagine how damaging they have been internally. When you are not fueling your body with healthy foods that are free of excessive processing, preservatives, and harsh chemicals, your brain does not operate optimally. You may feel sluggish or experience a common symptom known as "brain fog", you may feel unwell, anxious, or unable to concentrate. Irritability, frustration, and stress are reported in higher rates as a result of this, as well.

For your internal and external health, it is highly important that you are consuming a healthy diet. When you do, your entire body including your brain will operate at optimal levels and therefore you will be better able to engage in the mindfulness activities that will bring you the inner purification and happiness which you are seeking. It is important that you reduce the amount of unhealthy foods you ingest on a regular basis and start turning to healthier options more frequently.

Instant Gratification from Food

A large part of the eating experience is cooking your food. Understandably, sometimes you may prefer to visit a restaurant and sit down to someone else's cooking. However, you should consider the benefits that come from cooking your own meal. Aside from having control over what is in it and the flavors you will enjoy, you also increase your enjoyable experiences associated with eating. Your senses will become turned on and start to experience the food long before you start to eat it, and the overall process is a much more satisfying experience. You are likely to feel more fulfilled from your food.

Convenient and fast foods add to the 21st century problem that is a constant craving for instant gratification. Tactile marketing efforts show you that if you head to the convenient drive-through restaurant, you can enjoy a high-quality burger that would be just as good as if you were to make it on your own. However, we have already discussed how this is untrue and that you will actually end up eating something that looks nothing like the advertisement and tastes awful. And what's worse is it will be loaded with unwanted preservatives that make it even less healthy for you. Physically and mentally it creates a large problem.

Convenience foods contribute to the lack of sustained gratification and the cravings for instant gratification. We develop a greater desire to simply run and get it made for us in under 5 minutes, and if it's not done by then we sit in our cars and complain that our food is taking so long. Only, if we were to make it on our own at home it would take significantly longer. Though, it would taste infinitely better, too. The entire process of convenience food and fast food eliminate the value and pleasure associated with food and make it a mindless and highly stressful chore that we feel we must do in order to sustain our bodies. However, in many times we dread doing it because of the amount of stress we feel it brings into our lives.

Healthy Eating Alternatives

Listen, it makes sense why you may still want to enjoy the occasional fast food burger or sit down to restaurant meals. The point isn't to eliminate them one hundred percent. Rather, it is to realize that they are not a sustainable food source and that you should consider using healthier routes to eat your food. If you go the Middle Way on this, you will see that you can still enjoy these convenience food items, you simply don't need to enjoy them one hundred or even seventy-five percent of the time. Instead, you can enjoy them on a less frequent basis and feel more confident in knowing that you are making healthier food choices.

What exactly are healthier food choices, though? Well, you don't need to diet, that's for sure. Diets are short-term food intake changes that are not sustainable and frequently dissolve within' a few days to weeks. What you want to do is focus on having a total lifestyle shift that focuses more on the consumption of healthier foods. You should eat more leafy greens and fresh vegetables and fruits, as well as nuts on a regular basis for protein and all of the other added benefits that they have. You can also eat meat; however, don't consume massively large amounts. For example, one T-bone steak is generally enough meat to serve 2-3 people. Instead of indulging in one full one or the equivalent every single night or even for multiple meals a day, reduce yourself to simply enjoying the amount needed to acquire the protein and other nutrients you need to keep healthy.

When you are shopping, you should choose items that are non-gmo and certified organic. Whenever possible, choose grass-fed free-range options. These are ones that have been raised as close to the traditional farming practices as possible, and the companies tend to focus more on quality over quantity. As a result, you get higher quality produce that will provide you with greater nutritional value.

If you are busy, there are still ways to save time in your eating lifestyle. You don't need to prepare every meal from scratch three times a day every day of the week. Understanding that you are a modern person, you must also understand that your schedule may not allow for you to do that. What you can do, however, is prepare your meals in advance. Cut up your fruits and vegetables and place them in smaller single serving containers, make fresh homemade dips and put those in the containers as well. You can also prepare your meats and proteins a few days in advance to add to your meal preparations. The more you can do in advance if needed, the better. You are still gaining the valuable experience of food itself as you will see and experience the food during the creation process and therefore when the time comes to eat it you will be craving it and the satisfaction will be one that brings you sustainable gratification.

Eating does not have to be a chore that we accomplish as quick as possible. You do not need to be persuaded by mass media to consume foods that are unhealthy and that are ruining your body's health. Just because Western society views this as normal does not mean it is healthy nor optimal for your body. It is important that you listen in to what your body is telling you and that you nourish it in the healthiest ways possible. This way it will be able to serve you for years to come. You will experience significantly less stress, anxiety, depression, irritability and other mood disorders and physical health disorders as a result, as well.

Chapter Summary:

- Modern eating practices are not sustainable or healthy
- Convenient food eliminates the mindfulness and positive experiences associated with eating
- Processing methods and preservatives create unhealthy food items
- Unhealthy diets cause physical and mental illnesses that affect your mind and happiness
- The Middle Way means you can still occasionally indulge in convenient foods.
- Instant gratification obtained from food leads to more stress than anything else

Chapter 14: Consumerism

Mindfulness around the modern practices of consumerism has almost completely deteriorated. At one time, individuals would be thrilled if they were able to afford to purchase something new. They would discover an item they wanted, and then they would have to work to save up and make the money to afford it. When they could, the item would be enjoyed and would serve them and last for a long time. Now, however, we have achieved a consumerism mindset where we consistently want more. The instant gratification we experience with purchasing new items does not serve us for long, if at all. It has led us to a place where we no longer enjoy, cherish or appreciate the things that we acquire and use in our lives.

The Effects of Consumerism

Think about it, when you purchased your phone you were likely extremely excited when you first got it. You may have thought it was amazing because it was the top of the line model, or because it was better than your old phone. You cherished it for a few days, maybe even a few weeks. However, it quickly became something you disliked as you started to search for flaws within' it. When you realized someone else had a better phone or a newer model was released, you completely lost all appreciation for your phone. Now, instead of it being a source of joy and happiness, it is a source of pain. You suffer because you are no longer satisfied with your investment and you may even feel as though you are stuck with it if you entered one of the popular contracts or terms available through cell phone companies.

In an alternate scenario, let's think about your car, if you have one. On the day you brought it home, you were likely thrilled. You wanted to show it off and drive it around regularly, you were so proud of it and what it represented to you. It may have marked a new chapter in your life or been a physical token of your accomplishments. You were appreciative of your new car. In all likelihood, you washed it regularly and took good care of it. Once the novelty wore off, however, you stopped caring about your car. You washed it less frequently, you complained about it often, and you stopped showing appreciation for it and what it had to offer for you. The high-end stereo you were so excited about is now regarded as an outdated embarrassment. The leather seats that made you so happy about the car are now viewed as a flaw because they're either too hot or too cold. You start to notice all that it lacks, instead of appreciating it for what it is. It goes from being your token of success to your transportation of pain.

In the previous two scenarios, we are directly experiencing the outcome of instant gratification. This is what happens when we learn not to appreciate what we have but to constantly want the next best thing. A large part of this is the competition we are all in to be "the best". Only, no one will ever win because new things are always coming out, and therefore you will constantly be spending more money acquiring more things to achieve a status that is not actually attainable. In all actuality, you are trapping yourself within' what some people call "the rat race" and you are creating the perfect situation for suffering.

The Benefits of Consumerism

Despite the negative outcomes that can be associated with consumerism, it is important to refrain from regarding consumerism as an evil source. It isn't. Rather, it is the worldly perception that people carry that creates this appeal. When we stop to think about it, it is human nature to want to advance and invent. It exercises our creative abilities and allows us to expand our minds and awareness to consistently higher levels and achieve things that were once thought of as mere ideas and dreams. The industry that feeds consumerism is actually a beautiful piece of evidence of the ability humankind has to create anything they desire and bring it into the material world. It is important, however, that we learn to treat the industry with great respect and protect ourselves from the constant struggle to be the best.

The purpose of the consumerism industry primarily is to create "new stuff". Of course, money is needed to create more, so people market and advertise their items for sale. The funds then go back into creating more items. When people purchase certain items more than others, those items are what the inventors create more of, and the less popular items typically die off. It is a wonderful opportunity to see what actually serves our society and what is considered to be useless or unnecessary. When you understand this, you can understand the importance of the industry and the sales that take place within' it.

Instant Gratification and Consumerism

Unfortunately, many people feel as though they must have the "latest and greatest" in order to carry a desirable status in society. Simply put, this is completely false. In fact, a large majority of individuals would agree that they would prefer to hang out with an "outdated" person with a great personality versus a "trending" person who lacks any personality at all. The most important part of a person is their personality and their character when it comes to creating connections and being able to successfully socialize with others.

Often, people fail to recognize this however. Instead of noticing this and feeding their personality and being true to themselves, they purchase trendy items and attempt to make themselves appear "cool" or to have the "status" that everyone desires. If you were to look at people who carry this desirable "status" however, the majority of them are not ones who feed into the instant gratification areas of consumerism. It is rarely the ones who are consistently purchasing beyond their means and developing great stress and anxiety around their race to be better than everyone else. Instead, the ones who are most desired tend to be those who are extremely and perfectly happy with their lives as they are. It is the ones who are mindful of the value, quality, and appreciation they have for their belongings that are more desirable.

It is important to understand that the outward displays individuals show when they partake in the consumerism races directly correlate to their inward feelings about themselves and life. Their instant gratification sensations combined with frequent periods of suffering when they no longer appreciate their items directly shows how incapable they are of creating inner purity and peace. They lack happiness and therefore they attempt to purchase it through this status and these new items. They hope that the new items they acquire will bring them the happiness they seek. In truth, it brings them a fleeting feeling of it, or maybe even the idea of it. They often lack the actual deep experience of gratification and happiness, however, because it is not something you can purchase in the consumerism industry.

Mindful Consumerism

In order to protect yourself from this, it is important that you realize the way this instant gratification and need for status directly relates to mindfulness. When you are mindful of the way consumerism can create a downward spiral of insecurity and anxiety, you can then learn how to reverse engineer the process and make it more desirable and enjoyable for yourself. You give yourself the opportunity to become aware of these tendencies and behaviors and become more mindful over your belongings.

There are many ways that you can become more mindful about your consumerism practices. When you do so, you will find that you discover greater enjoyment from your purchases and that they bring you happiness, satisfaction, and fulfillment for much longer than when you were a serial shopper. These methods are simple ways that you can instill in your life that make it easy for you to become more mindful over your belongings and refrain from the suffering that people associate with their consumerism purchases.

Dissolve Attachment to Old Belongings

The most important thing you should do before bringing new items into your house is to consider the old items you already own. You will want to learn to dissolve your attachments to old items. Simply because it brought you joy in the past does not mean that it will continue to bring you joy in the present or the future. If it is something that is not bringing you joy in the present moment to the fullest degree, or that hasn't brought you joy in recent times, it is likely time to let it go. Often, when you let things go you can give other people the opportunity to experience the joy associated with the item if you choose to donate it or sell it. Alternatively, you may wish to put it in the garbage. Either way, you will want to learn to dissolve your attachment to old things.

When you dissolve your attachments and give yourself permission to let go of things that you no longer use, you give yourself the opportunity to clear up space within' your home. A large part of stress that is brought on by consumerism is that it leads to chaotic and messy living quarters that eliminate the amount of joy you would experience when bringing new things into your home. Instead of enjoying said new item, you would likely feel more stressed because there was now more clutter in your home. If you were to first clear space for the new items, then you would have the room physically and emotionally to enjoy them more thoroughly.

Dissolve Attachment to New Stuff

In addition to dissolving your attachments to old things, you need to dissolve it to new things as well. Understand that purchasing new things will not always bring you what you are seeking and that often it will actually bring the exact opposite. If you purchase things for a specific happiness you are chasing, realize that you often will be working in direct reverse of the happiness you actually desire. Purchasing items for pure inner happiness will not return said result. Instead, it will create a situation where you affirm that you are not capable of instantly satisfying a need for pure happiness or a certain status, and you will end up feeling worse.

When you are purchasing new things, you need to ensure that you are purchasing it for the right reasons. Understanding why you want it and how it will serve you will assist you in making wise decisions that will make it easier for you to make your purchases and feel joy and satisfaction from them, instead of guilt and suffering.

Consider How It Will Serve You

When you are investing in something, consider exactly how that item will serve you. What about it makes it valuable to you? Are you purchasing it for the ability to say you own it? Or are you purchasing it because it offers many features that will make it usable and worthwhile to you for a long time? It is wise that you do not rush through these answers. Those who fly through them with "yes" will often discover the true answer was no, but they failed to truly decipher why they wanted said item. Ensure that you take the time to deeply understand what is attracting you to said item and really consider what it will bring you in your life.

Invest Wisely

In addition to considering the service the item will have in your life, consider your financial situation. Are you investing more than you have to invest? Are you going into debt to acquire said item? If so, you need to be even more cautious about how said item is going to enhance your life. If you were to go into debt and realize in two months that it did not have what you desired to acquire, you are going to feel double the amount of suffering when you consider said item. You will realize that you are now spending money on something you own but do not like. It is worse than if you were to spend the money you had on it only to find out that you did not like it.

Even if you are spending it through a debit account and are not going into debt, you still need to consider how it is going to affect your finances. You may not be going into debt directly or even financially, but in one way or another it may lead you there. Ensure that you take the time and you act from a firm financial foundation so that your new investment does not lead to excessive suffering.

Take The Time to Enjoy Your New Items

In a consumerist society, it is common to be a serial purchaser. In one day you may find it easy to spend $100 or even several hundreds of dollars on new items. When you get them home, you may find that you only actually like one or two and that you are not really using the rest. It is not necessarily that you don't like them, but perhaps you don't like them as much. Alternatively, you may be too overwhelmed with all of the new items and therefore you pick the most convenient ones and the rest are forgotten.

When you are investing in new items and purchasing them, space it out. Purchase new things gradually and take the time to truly enjoy and integrate new items into your life. When you do this, each one will serve a strong purpose and you will feel ongoing satisfaction. Instead of spending all of your spare cash on payday and being broke between checks, you will be able to acquire new things slowly throughout the time between paychecks or even longer, and you will be able to invest more time in actually enjoying them. This eliminates the instant gratification of the consumerism market and increases the sustainable gratification you experience when you are spending money. It will often put you in a healthier financial situation, as well, as you will learn to decipher what you truly want and what you like but don't necessarily want or need.

Chapter Summary:

- Consumerism isn't evil
- Creativity and invention is healthy for human advancement and expansion
- Unhealthy consumerist perceptions can create stress, anxiety, and suffering
- Dissolving attachments to old and new things can clear up a lot of emotional baggage
- Healthy consuming habits can increase the joy you experience with your new items

Chapter 15: Stress

Stress is one of the biggest forms of suffering that people endure in life and in modern times the stress we encounter comes from a wide range of sources. Virtually everywhere in our life is enhanced with stress, particularly when we nurture the instant gratification areas of our lives. Our constant need to have more stuff and to fulfill those desires immediately leads us to a number of stressors that we, as a society, are lead to endure. This largely deviates away from mindfulness practices and makes it harder for us to achieve inner purification and happiness.

Throughout this entire book, you have grown to understand the danger of instant gratification and the amount of emotional baggage that it carries. Whenever we push to be instantly gratified, we find ourselves encountering infinitely more stressors than we would otherwise. We find stress in driving, in waiting, in watching. We find stress in paying for things we can't afford, and in standing in lines for things we already know are ours. We find stress in parking, in talking to others, and in sharing with our friends. Ultimately, every area of our life that is intended to bring us joy is infused with stress in some format.

There are a number of ways that stress can affect your body and mind, none of which can be considered healthy when it is endured in the high amounts that we face. When we are faced with high stress levels for a short period of time, we tend to experience symptoms such as tightness in the chest, headaches, irritability, weight gain or loss, aches and pains, and a number of other symptoms. When we are faced with high stress levels for a long period of time, as we are often faced with in the 21st century, it can lead to even larger problems, sometimes even fatal. You may experience asthma, obesity, accelerated aging, heart attack or heart disease, gastrointestinal problems, diabetes, or depression and anxiety. The number of ways that prolonged stress exposure can deeply affect us are almost infinite. While these are the most common methods, there are many other ways you can be affected, as well.

Stress isn't always negative. Just as everything in life, not enough stress is potentially dangerous and too much stress is definitely dangerous. When we lead a life with zero stress, we run the risk of falling into stagnant patterns. We do not feel the need or urge to make necessary changes in our life and so we end up finding a stale situation. In healthy levels, stress encourages change. And change itself is vital. When you are in a healthy stress management system, you give yourself the ability to make changes without experiencing health ailments directly related to that stress. You learn to listen to your body and respect your stress mechanism and take action when your body tells you that it is time to. In doing so, you gain the ability to respect your body's signals and make mandatory changes in your life.

Mindfulness and stress work hand-in-hand. When you are more mindful, you are less stressed. Likewise, when you are less stressed, you are more mindful. How you will achieve the perfect balance is largely based on what your current average stress level is in life. The best way to find out is to consider how you have been dealing with stress lately. The more stressed you are, the more mindful you are going to need to become over your stress and therefore the harder it may be for you to achieve this mindfulness in the beginning. If you are largely stressed to the point that this is your primary problem, this should be your main focus when you are learning to eliminate stress in your life.

Lowering your stress levels to a healthy place requires dedication, persistence, and focus. You will not be able to rid yourself of stress all in one go, nor will you be able to ever rid yourself of it entirely. Reducing your stress to a healthy level allows you to regain respect for stress and the ways it can enhance your life when you perceive it as an effective and powerful tool to encourage change. You may be curious as to how you can start reducing your stress in order to practice mindfulness more effectively and lead a happier life. The truth is, there are many ways. Later in this book, you are going to learn specific practices to achieve mindfulness, but right now you will gain an insight on some of the ways you will be able to do this.

The best way to handle stress using the methods you have learned in this book is to consider the Four Noble Truths. If you will remember, they are: suffering exists, suffering arises from attachment to desires, suffering ceases when attachment to desires ceases, and freedom from suffering is possible by the Eightfold Path. Knowing this, you can figure out a powerful way to take action and make a change in your life so that you can reduce your stress to a healthy amount and learn to respect your stress better.

The first truth, that suffering exists, is clear when we are highly stressed. The stress in and of itself is a form of suffering, and if you have been experiencing it for a prolonged amount of time then you are suffering in a large way from your stress. It can be damaging and dangerous and you need to learn to first figure out how you can honestly recognize it as suffering. You can do this by becoming mindful over the times that you experience stress. When you are experiencing stress, you should open yourself up to being aware of this and mindful of the situation itself. What brought on the stress? What caused you to feel it and how do you feel as a result? What does stress make you feel inside? Outside? How does stress affect your life? Gaining a strong mindful practice around stress and how it affects you is important. You should take some time to reflect on this before you move on to the next step.

You may feel compelled to rush through your mindfulness practice when it comes to identifying stress. However, it is not beneficial to do so. Of course, you are going to have answers that arise immediately to tell you about your stress. Ideally, you should write these down. Then, the more you linger on the questions, the more answers you will gain from them. This is because you are experiencing the symptoms of stress in the immediate moment, which means that you are emotionally charged and you are only thinking about that which serves your stress. When you give yourself time to relax slightly or at least detach from the situation itself, you give yourself a better ability to answer the questions more thoroughly and gain more insight on them. This insight is what will assist you in making the right changes in the next steps.

The second Noble Truth is that suffering arises as a result of attachment. Whenever you are attached to something, whether it is an object, a person, a situation, a perceived social status or otherwise, you will suffer. You cannot possibly refrain from suffering because you have attachment and anytime you feel said attachment is compromised, you are going to suffer. With the constant fluctuations and changes in life combined with the mark of existence that states impermanence is inevitable, you are going to certainly feel suffering. It is likely that you know that the attachment you are feeling will terminate eventually, and your denial about that is what causes the suffering.

If you are experiencing stress in your life and you have taken the time to become mindful over the question "why?" and you have thoughtfully answered this question, then you can likely identify what the attachment is. Is it to your job? To a social status? To a person? Are you attached to a specific emotion or sensation? When you identify this attachment, you give yourself a better ability to deal with the stress you encounter. This means that you have a better chance to eradicate the excessive stress levels and bring yourself back down to the healthier levels. It is inevitable that the stress you are experiencing is the result of an attachment you have to something in your life. The sooner you work to identify that attachment, the easier it will be to reduce your stress levels.

The third Noble Rule is that suffering ceases when attachment ceases. When you realize this and you know what your attachment is, then you know that you must dissolve that attachment in order to dissolve your stress. Your stress has risen to inform you of this stress and what it has brought to your life, and you must then address your stress by eliminating the attachment. There are many ways that you can eliminate attachments, the exact method you will use will be largely based on what your specific situation is. You may have to dissolve a friendship, or a standard you are carrying that your body is telling you is not achievable by you at this time. You may have to dissolve your attachment to a social status or to a certain emotion, and then you will be able to eradicate the suffering you are experiencing through stress.

Dissolving attachment doesn't always mean to get rid of the specific item or person your attachment is associated to. Sometimes, it is dissolving your attachment to the high expectations you have around said item or person. When you do this, you gain freedom from the attachment while still giving yourself the ability to live a life with said item or person present. Instead of suffering in the way you once did, though, you will now be liberated from that suffering and you will feel more peace and happiness around something that once brought you that severe suffering in the form of stress.

The fourth and final Noble Rule is that freedom of suffering is possible by the Eightfold Path. When you are mindfully following the Eightfold Path, you give yourself the ability to free yourself from this suffering and all suffering that may be brought about in the future by similar attachments. The Eightfold Path contains eight methods you can use in order to eradicate your suffering and dissolve attachments. You can then learn to have a healthy relationship with your stress and use it as a tool to propel you forward in life, instead of an emotion that brings about a great deal of baggage through suffering and stress in your life.

Stress is not something that needs to be regarded as dangerous. Instead, it is an emotion that informs us that change needs to be made in order to allow us to survive in peace. In modern times, however, we often fail to form healthy relationships with stress and therefore we see it as a means of suffering and pain. We do not realize that stress means we require change in our lives; instead, we see it as some evil emotional sensation we carry that has no purpose other than to cause suffering in our lives. When we view stress in this unhealthy way, we are lead to a point where we no longer benefit from stress and what it has to offer us. Instead, it brings about significant emotional baggage, physical and emotional symptoms, and a large amount of suffering.

Even among our highly stressful lives, we have the ability to change the way stress affects us and start viewing it in a healthier way. When we take the time to identify each stressor and take into consideration what is causing it and what our attachments are that are causing suffering, then we give ourselves the ability to make powerful and meaningful changes. As a result, we are able to liberate ourselves to freedom and feel empowered and happy within' our lives. Then, we open ourselves up to the ability to achieve inner purity and propel ourselves towards nirvana.

Chapter Summary:

- Stress is a healthy emotion that we often view as emotional baggage due to our high levels of it
- When we view stress as suffering, it is because of an attachment we have
- Identifying the attachment and dissolving it liberates us to freedom
- When we achieve this freedom we learn to open ourselves up to more of it
- Healthy stress levels encourage us to make necessary changes in life

Part 4: Mindfulness Practice

Until now, you have learned numerous powerful teachings to invoke thought and encourage you to consider your mindfulness practice on a deeper level. You have been encouraged to understand the greatest depths of your mind and ask the questions that will draw you into a mindful state and help you understand yourself and how you can truly become mindful as opposed to just self-aware.

Buddhist teachings have a powerful way of teaching us how we can question ourselves in our lives in a way that can draw us towards the answers that will bring us inner purity, peace and happiness. By now, you likely have a strong idea on the areas you need to become more mindful in. You perhaps have discovered some of your biggest sufferings and how you can relieve yourself of those pains and draw yourself forward into freedom and liberation from that suffering and closer to nirvana. The next step is to learn exactly how you can deepen your mindfulness practice on a regular basis and really reinforce it in your life. You can do so by having a strong mindfulness routine that you practice on a regular basis. Preferably, you will be practicing your mindfulness on a daily basis as frequently as possible.

The next part of your mindfulness journey you need to learn and focus on is the development of that routine. You need to learn exactly how you can develop a mindfulness routine that will enable you to establish a solid foundation for your mindfulness and grow from there. When you learn how you can create your own unique mindfulness practice, you will then be able to powerfully strengthen and reinforce your mindfulness journey. You will find that it becomes even easier for you to detach yourself from suffering and that you will draw yourself closer and closer to happiness, peace, and purity with each step you take.

Remember, the process to mindfulness is gradual and for many, it takes a lifetime. Sometimes, it may even take several lifetimes. The best thing that you can do is discover what you can do right now in order to establish a powerful mindfulness practice that is going to allow you to achieve higher levels of freedom, peace, and happiness on a daily basis. As you do this, you will begin to feel better than ever and you will draw yourself nearer to the ability to truly experience inner purity.

Chapter 16: Meditation

In Buddhist traditions, meditation is a practice that is done on a daily basis. And, for good reason. In fact, many people all over the world whether they are religious, traditional, or simply spiritual or otherwise prefer to have a daily meditation routine. Meditation has a powerful ability to assist you in clearing your mind and sitting with your thoughts, feelings, and energies. When you meditate, you are able to reduce your stress levels, gain clarity on your life and feelings, and draw yourself in deeper to your own inner workings and a greater understanding of self. In doing so, you give yourself the ability to become even more mindful over yourself and what you can do in order to encourage your life to reflect more of what you desire from it.

Benefits of Meditation

Meditating brings with it a number of wonderful benefits, especially when it comes to mindfulness. As you have already learned, it is a major help when it comes to eliminating and reducing stress in your life. You also gain a greater sense of self-awareness which is crucial when you are developing your mindfulness practice. Another way meditation helps is that it has been shown to assist people in regulating their emotions and developing a stronger emotional intelligence rating. This is a powerful way to help you view emotions as triggers that tell you how your body need to be nurtured so that you can care for it in a way that supports it perfectly. Those who meditate are also known to have reduced symptoms of anxiety, depression, and PTSD. As well, they learn faster and are able to absorb information easier. Finally, when you meditate and you work together with your emotions in your body through mindfulness practices, you give yourself the ability to change how you naturally respond to certain situations and triggers. You can alter your fight-or-flight mode "settings" and you can learn to enforce behavior you would rather experience instead of behaving in a way that is automatic to your situation or trigger.

Ultimately, meditating is a wonderful way to exercise and strengthen your brain and your mind. There are so many benefits that arise from meditating on an emotional and physical level, so that alone should be reason enough to want to start meditating in your daily life! When you are able to reap all of the benefits from having a regular meditation practice, you give yourself the opportunity to powerfully change your life through mindfulness and the ability to control your mind in a way that empowers you. It is important to realize, however, that meditation is not a practice we use to achieve happiness. Rather, it is a practice to learn about the laws of impermanence. If you use meditation to achieve happiness you will not achieve it each time and suffer as a result. Like anything, happiness is impermanent and meditation is not a practice that can guarantee its return. Instead, use it as a practice to recognize the impermanence and come to peace with the present circumstances.

"Meditation brings wisdom; lack of meditation leaves ignorance. Know well what leads you forward and what holds you back, and choose the path that leads to wisdom."

-Buddha

The Science of Meditation

Although the Buddha likely knew nothing about the science of meditation, he knew deeply about the wisdom that it could bring you. And as you know, wisdom is the best way to work through your inner world and lead yourself to happiness, peace, and purity. When you are wise in life, you are able to make decisions and choices that are not emotionally charged, but rather logically based. You can make the decisions that are most important for your development and spiritual growth, and refrain from making decisions from emotional baggage. You also give yourself the ability to alleviate the emotional baggage you may feel would come with doing the "right" thing.

Now, several years later, we have science around how the Tibetan monks were actually benefitted from meditation and its powerful effects. The research that has been completed on their minds has proven that it increases their attention skills and shifts their awareness. They tend to have two developed networks within' their brains: the extrinsic and the intrinsic networks. The latter of which is also known as the default network. The extrinsic network that experienced meditation practitioners have is activated when they are partaking in external activities such as drinking something or playing a sport. The intrinsic network is activated with reflection and anything that involves the individual paying attention to their emotions and inner self. An important thing to note is that the two rarely function at full rate at the same time, and therefore you are not likely to be able to develop your own intrinsic network when you are being activated by the extrinsic one.

How Long to Meditate

Many people who do not practice meditation on a regular basis believe that it requires hours and hours of your time every day. The truth is, for modern people an optimal meditation time is between 15-20 minutes, and you gain more from it by having a few shorter meditation sessions during the day than you do if you were to have one long one each day. The most commonly suggested times for meditation is first thing in the morning when you are freshly awake and then last thing at night before you go to bed. When you meditate in the morning, you give yourself the opportunity to wake up and set your mind to be in the space that you want it to be in for the remainder of your day.

Alternatively, when you meditate at night before bed, you allow yourself to shed the experiences of the day and draw yourself into a relaxed state before you fall asleep so that you can have a deeper and more restful sleep.

You may think that meditation is going to be hard. How can you simply close your eyes and acquire wisdom? The truth is, it is easier than you may think, and the wisdom is not something you chase but rather something you are given. When you meditate on a regular basis, you will find it becomes second nature and that you can enter a meditative state quite easily. As a result, you may even find that your stress management on-the-go is much better, too!

How to Meditate

To get started with meditating, there are some things you will want to consider before you close your eyes. There are many ways to increase your meditation practice by first making your surroundings more calming and welcoming. Some people prefer to have a blanket around them. Some prefer to sit, and others prefer to lie down. Some prefer to sit in a chair with their feet on the floor, and others prefer to sit on the ground with their legs crossed and a small pillow beneath them. Others still prefer no pillow at all and would rather sit directly on the floor. Of course, if you are meditating you will want to sit wherever is most comfortable for you since your body will need to be comfortable in order for you to go into your mind for a short while.

For some people, a comfortable seating arrangement is all that they require in order to meditate effectively. For others, they prefer to have aromatherapy, calm lighting, and soft music on in the background. There is no right or wrong way to arrange your meditation space, so long as you are able to find comfort within' it and that it is easy for you to go into your mind for a short period of time without feeling as though you need to move your body or like you are becoming uncomfortable. You should not have to worry about your body at all while you meditate, it should be simple and relaxing for you.

When you are ready and your surroundings are comfortable enough for you, you can go ahead and sit or lie down in the position that is most comfortable. Then, you can start meditating! To do so, you will first want to become mindful of your surroundings and your body. Before you close your eyes, take a look at what is around you. Notice things that you may not notice otherwise, and notice what feelings or emotions come up when you take the time to see these things. Don't judge yourself, just look on. When you are ready, start becoming mindful of your body. What can you notice about how your body feels? How does that make you feel, if it brings up any emotions or feelings within' yourself? Again, don't judge this, just simply notice it.

As thoughts come into your mind, recognize them, sit with them, and then let them pass. Don't dwell on them, simply regard them and let them go. When you start to notice that your awareness on the present moment has become lost to your inner thoughts, return your attention to the present moment and start noticing what you can become aware of. When you're ready, close your eyes and do the same. What can you feel within' you? What do you notice about those feelings? Take the time to really sit with all of the feelings and emotions that come up with you, but then effortlessly let them roll away as you move on and bring your awareness back to the present moment.

The most important part of meditation is that it is intended to bring stress-relief which you cannot achieve if you are judging yourself or becoming angry because you find your mind is wandering more than you desire for it to. It is crucial that you are kind to your mind and your thoughts and that you do not take any harsh or emotionally charged stances towards anything that you are experiencing inside or outside of yourself. When you are able to objectively acknowledge the present moment, you give yourself the ability to truly enjoy it.

Body Scan Meditation

For some people, this does not feel like enough information to meditate for a full fifteen to twenty minutes. If you find that is you, then you may wish to follow the guide below on how you can do a basic body scan and bring yourself into a deepened state of relaxation. Doing this will make your meditation practice easier since you will know exactly what you need to do to master it. Body scans are a wonderful way to gain awareness on your body and become mindful over anything that may be bothering you that you may not notice in your regularly busy life.

Sit in Your Comfortable Spot

Now that you have created the space for your comfortable meditation, you will want to settle into it. Whether you chose a chair, your bed, a pillow or the floor, get yourself situated in a way that is comfortable and prepare to meditate. Take your time and make sure you are truly comfortable. If you need to, shake out your excess energy just before sitting down or getting comfortable so that you don't feel a significant urge to fidget or move around while you are meditating. Doing this will make it easier for you to sit still for longer.

Become Aware of Your Legs

When you are ready, take the time to notice your legs. You can become aware of how they are placed, how you may be able to comfort them more, and what they feel like in general. If something is bothering you within' your legs or feet, you can make a mental note now and when you are done meditating you can be sure to take action to make it better. Notice things such as how the air feels against your legs and how they feel rested against whatever your chosen seating is. Take your time on these awareness processes so you can truly feel what everything feels like and bring your total attention to your body.

Straighten Your Upper Body

Once you have noticed your legs, now move your awareness to your upper body. Can you identify any sensations within' it? Straighten your back and stretch the crown of your head towards the sky as you elongate your spine. Take the time to develop an awareness of the sensations you experience such as tight muscles, the clothes against your skin, or anything else that may be creating sensations for your upper body. If you notice anything uncomfortable or out of the normal, be sure to take a mental note and when you're done you can take appropriate action to alleviate your symptoms.

Become Aware of Your Arms

When you are ready, draw your awareness into your arms. Start to notice your shoulders and then draw your awareness all the way down your arms and into your fingertips. Once again, take note on all of the sensations you feel and whether or not anything in either arm feels unwell or tense. Draw your awareness into all things that are bringing any sensation to your arms: the air, your clothes, a blanket, or anything else that may be touching them. You may notice that when you are paying attention to a certain area of your body it develops a different sensation or a warmth to it that is not otherwise present when your awareness is elsewhere, take notice of that.

Become Aware of Your Head

When you are ready, bring your awareness up into your neck and your head. Take the time to go through all areas of your neck, head, and face. Think about the way your throat, shoulders, neck, scalp, chin, cheeks, forehead and ears feel. What can you notice about these? How does your hair feel against your skin? Do you feel the air against your skin? Is there anything else that you can become aware of? If you notice anything is tense or unwell, take a note so you can take action later.

Send a Loving Intention

Although the purpose of meditation is not necessarily to heal, you can take a moment to set a loving intention for your practice. If you have noticed tension or discomfort anywhere within' your body, you may wish to send your loving intention towards that sensation so that you can become mindful over it and do what you can to alleviate it. Otherwise, you may simply wish to set a loving intention for your entire practice in general. Once you have set your intention, let it go.

Soften Your Gaze

Now that you are completely present and aware of your body, take the time to let your eyelids lower and your eyes close. If this is not comfortable for you to completely close your eyes, you may prefer to simply allow them to become lazy and focus indirectly on something around you. Allow your eyes to relax in whatever way feels most comfortable for you, and you will be just fine.

Become Aware of Your Breath

When you are ready, draw your awareness into your breath. Feel the air as it fills your lungs, and feel it draw back out as well. You may wish to practice yogic breathing for something to focus on and as a means to deeply relax yourself. To do so, you want to fill your diaphragm, lungs and throat, then empty the air from your throat, lungs and diaphragm. Do so slowly and intentionally. Allow the air to come in your nose and gently let it rush out between your lips. Do whatever feels most relaxing for you when it comes to your breath, and keep your awareness on it. Pay attention to all of the sensations your body has when you are breathing deeply. Some people who are laying down may wish to bring their hands over their abdomen and feel each breath as it enters and exits the body. That is completely okay and you can do so if it feels comfortable for you. Some people find that this makes it easier to maintain an awareness of the body and the breath itself since they are physically feeling it with their hands.

When Your Mind Wanders, Gently Draw It Back

Your mind will inevitably wander when you are meditating. After all, we are mental beings who have constant thoughts. That is why you should be aware that meditation is not about completely eliminating the wandering thoughts. Rather, it is about becoming mindful about when the thought comes into your mind, recognizing it, and letting it go. Whenever you realize your mind is wandering too far or you have lost the presence within' your body, you can simply draw your awareness back to your breath. Be gentle and kind when you are drawing your awareness back, as you have no need to worry about these wandering thoughts since they are completely normal and expected.

Be Kind to Yourself

Throughout the entire process of meditation, you should be kind to yourself. Meditation is not a practice that we should compete in or that we can do "good" or "bad" in. As long as you are meditating, you are doing well with it. There is no standard to hold yourself to or no rules to strictly stand by. You can do whatever feels most comfortable for you and stay confident in the fact that it means you are doing it right. Whenever you notice your mind wanders, do not become resentful or angry with yourself. Do not allow yourself to venture into a state of stress, frustration or anxiety when you feel as though your mind or body does not respond or react the way you believe it should. Instead, be kind to yourself, your mind and your body. When you notice it is doing something you prefer it wouldn't, such as leaving the presence of the moment, simply draw it back kindly and gently.

When You're Ready, Come Back to The Room

You can meditate for as short or as long as you desire. If you are comfortable with focusing on your breath, you may prefer to just stay in that moment for a while. If you are feeling as though you are done with your meditation session, you can simply bring your awareness back to the room and open your eyes or return your awareness to your surroundings.

You may find that you only meditate for about 5-10 minutes at first. In fact, you may find that your own meditation practice never lasts longer than that. If that is what you discover, that is completely okay and you have nothing to worry about. As previously mentioned, frequent shorter practices are better than longer practices or ones that are nonexistent! Alternatively, you may find that your mindfulness practice lasts longer than 20 minutes, maybe even above half an hour or closer to an hour or even longer. That is completely fine as well! Even more, you may find that the length of time you meditate fluctuates each time you actually meditate. Once again, this is completely normal and okay. The most important thing is that you set aside time on a regular basis to accomplish your meditation practice and bring your awareness to the present moment and your breath.

Alternative Meditation for Mindfulness

In addition to actual structured meditation sessions, there are other ways that you can practice the mindfulness associated with meditation and develop your intrinsic network that we previously discovered. In fact, a large portion of the foundation of mindfulness is developed within' the practices that develop your intrinsic network. You can develop it through regularly checking in with your body as you go about your daily activities. For example, when you are driving, walking, or cooking supper you can check in with your body and the sensations you are experiencing. You can take the time to notice everything you are experiencing within' you and what your body feels like. You can notice what the smells around you are and what you are hearing. As well, you can notice what you feel and the sensations against your skin on your body. If you are eating, take the time to notice what you are tasting and the texture of the food in every bite. How are they different from one another? You can do these tune-ins on a regular basis to become aware of the present moment and draw your attention back to what you are doing. It is important that you are always present in the moment as much as possible.

When you meditate and you objectively view the emotions and sensations that arise within' you, you will likely find that you notice things you did not notice otherwise. As well, often times you will draw new conclusions that you were not aware of in your regular busy life. Meditation gives us the space to develop a mindful awareness of ourselves, our lives and our thoughts. We are able to recognize our surroundings, our feelings and emotions, and the thoughts that appear to be affecting us most in the present. Knowing all of this, we are able to draw conclusions that often assist us through these situations, or simply allow us to experience the emotion and let it go.

There are many benefits to meditating and many reasons why you should do it on a regular basis. If you still struggle to meditate in the beginning, despite having your surroundings arranged and the guide on what you should do during your practice, you may wish to use guided meditations. Guided meditations are audio tracks that have been created by others' who meditate that enable you to follow their voice and be guided through your meditation experience as you actively do it. Some people discover this is a wonderful way for them to start meditating because it teaches them what to do. Once they learn what the meditative state actually feels like, then they give themselves the ability to meditate easier on their own without the guidance.

Remember, whatever feels right for you is what you should do. There are no strict rules on how one should meditate or what one must do or think about when they are meditating. Instead, you simply do what feels comfortable and right for you. Then, when you are done, you carry on with your daily life. As long as you are doing what feels relaxing and beneficial to you, you are going to be able to benefit from the many wonderful outcomes of meditation. That is a given.

Chapter Summary:

- Meditation is a powerful way to achieve mindfulness
- Regular short sessions are more powerful than fewer long sessions
- Meditating does not have to be hard for you to do
- Meditation helps eliminate emotional baggage and other attachments to suffering
- People who meditate frequently tend to bear more wisdom than others
- Alternative meditation allows you to "check-in" on a regular basis and develop your practice further

Chapter 17: The Four Principles

There are four principles that you should include in your mindfulness practice on a regular basis. These are ways of being for you to become aware of and enforce them as regularly as you possibly can. In doing so, you create an easier space for you to be mindful in all of your activities. Being mindful when you are meditating is easy: your body is still and you are able to think about what you are doing and relax. When you are actively engaged in your day, however, it can take a little more work to become mindful. These four principles will help you.

Frankness

When you are frank, you are portraying the characteristics of being open and honest. A large part of mindfulness is being able to embrace frankness and embody it in your daily life. Honesty and being open is the best way to convey what is on your mind and live in your truth. It gives you the upper hand when it comes to relieving yourself of emotional baggage and living a life that is mindful and pure. It prevents you from holding on to things that should be expressed and gives you the opportunity to clear your mind and lead from a place of peace.

Being frank can be hard, especially when you fear your truth may hurt the feelings of others or cause unwanted results that may be painful. If you are feeling this way and your honesty is bringing you stress, you should pay attention to what your attachments are in life. You may be experiencing the attachment to people pleasing and that in itself is causing you to be stressed out and unwell. Alternatively, you may be stressed about losing your job or something that you feel is important to you. Regardless, you should recall the existence of impermanence. When you speak your truth, you may experience some pain as a result but the peace you experience will outweigh that. As well, any pain or peace you experience will be impermanent, but at least the peace will draw you to a higher place where you can further seek internal peace. Pain will keep you shrunken and sheltered away and cause you to continue suffering for a prolonged period of time over something that is generally not worth suffering over.

Even if you struggle with it now, you should learn to live your life in complete honesty by being frank. When you are confident in your honesty, you can become confident that the outcome will always benefit you in one way or another, even if it is merely by shedding emotional baggage. It is important that you learn to be completely honest. You should not work to flatter others or be sly or slick in any way. There is no reason for you to avoid responsibilities or evade blame. Accept responsibility for what you do and what you must do, and be open and willing to accept criticism from others around you.

When you are frank, you accept things as they are. You admit to yourself and the world that you are human and you make human mistakes. You admit that you have emotions and that you desire for them to be heard when necessary. You eliminate the need for you to seem above others or better in any way. Instead, you are honest and modest about who you are. You are true about who you are, what you do, what belongs to you and what doesn't. When you are criticized or given advice, you accept it and apply it when and where necessary and let go of anything else that does not serve you. There is no reason to lie or evade anything. Simply accept things as they are.

Simplicity

Another way to maintain mindfulness is to open yourself up to simplicity. Many people in modern times are accomplishing this through a lifestyle known as "minimalism" which ultimately means that you are reducing your belongings to only that which serves you or brings you great joy. When something no longer fulfills either purpose, it is rehomed or thrown away. There are many ways you can be simple in life, whether you choose to be a minimalist or not. You are not required to turn to extreme minimalism to enjoy a simplistic life, nor are you required to really turn to one at all. However, when you start leading a more mindful life with simplicity, it is likely that you will naturally start living a more minimalistic life as a result.

There are a number of areas in your life that you can simplify to make easier. You can simplify one or all of these areas, though the more you simplify the easier your mindfulness will practice will be.

Wardrobe

In your external life, you may wish to simplify your wardrobe. Rather than having a number of articles of clothes that only go together with one or two things and thus having an enormous amount of stuff, you may wish to reduce to only having a few things. Doing so reduces the amount of stress and responsibility you have associated with your wardrobe. It makes it easier for you to get dressed and easier for you to manage your wardrobe. As a result, you will feel more liberation and freedom in your wardrobe.

Home

As with your wardrobe, you can also simplify your home. Eliminate and reduce clutter and seriously consider letting go of everything that doesn't serve you or bring you joy. It is important that your external world, particularly your home, is one that reflects the internal world you are trying to create. Since mindfulness is largely about simplicity, you will want to create a more simplistic home. Instead of having something on every surface or clutter in every corner, eliminate things and create a space that reflects clarity and peace. Then, you will realize that your mind will follow suit.

Entertainment

Another way that you can simplify your life is through entertainment. In this generation, it is common to constantly look outward for entertainment and spend enormous amounts of money and energy on being entertained. We head to movies, live events, amusement parks, parties and other locations that can bring about entertainment. However, it can also bring about emotional baggage. Especially if we are using entertainment as a means to run away from emotions we are experiencing when we are alone and not having such a large amount of fun. You can still go out and have fun in these ways, there is no need to completely eliminate them. Instead, you should simply become more intentional about what you do, where you go, and how you spend your money, time and energy on your outings. When you do so, you will create the space for infinitely more peace in your mind.

Indulgence

You previously read about consumerism, and here is where you should really think about it. There is no need to over indulge in things or spend money merely because you have it. Instead, you should learn to simplify how you indulge and spend your money. When you are indulging in consumable items like food, consider what you are indulging in and how much. If you take your time, a small bit here and there is completely fine. The same goes for purchasing items, take your time and purchase slowly, intentionally and thoughtfully. The more intention and simplicity you put into your indulging behaviors, the easier it will be for you to indulge. You will not have to worry so much about what you are spending or clutter you are collecting because everything you purchase serves a purpose, either by bringing you joy or fulfilling a need.

Activities

In modern times, we are a very go-go-go society. We often find ourselves doing what is known as "over-exertion" leading to higher stress levels, reduced alertness and awareness, and other unwanted emotional baggage. When we take the time to relax more, such as by meditating or simply becoming aware of the present moment and reducing our activities, we give ourselves the space to further increase our mindfulness. We allow ourselves to remove from the external world and spend some time in the internal world, which is equally as important. We give ourselves the space and ability to gain wisdom, clarity, and mindfulness about our lives and our circumstances. Then, our personal development grows and so, too, does our mind.

Society is wordy. We send instant messages, share status updates, talk on the phones, chat in person, and gossip an enormous amount. We are constantly talking and communication through one way or another. It can lead to a large deal of emotional baggage. We find that we are gossiping about others and being unkind in our words on a regular basis, even when we try not to be. We find that we often say things that needn't be said merely for the purpose of speaking or being heard. If we feel we are not understood, we explain ourselves excessively to attempt to gain the understanding of others. In doing so, it can be highly exhausting and bring about a large amount of emotional baggage. Essentially, we look outward for affirmation and appreciation rather than inward.

When you are speaking, be simplistic in your words. Say only what needs to be said, and attempt to refrain from saying too much. There is no need to update your status every few hours, send text messages every few minutes, or talk simply because someone is present. Instead, take the time to enjoy the silent presence of others and the silent presence of yourself. See what you can learn from the silence and observation, as opposed to what you miss when you are constantly communicating and talking. When you are communication, speak with intention and purpose, and listen with the intention to listen, not the intention to answer.

Thought

Mindfulness is the practice of developing intention in your thoughts and mental presence so it makes sense that you would want to bring simplicity into your thoughts. When you do, you give yourself the ability to think with greater intention. You allow yourself the opportunity to refrain from excessive and obsessive thinking that may lead you into areas that bring on unwanted emotional baggage. You also give yourself space to let go of the thoughts that don't serve you and focus more intently on the ones that do. Do not evade thoughts, simply let them go. As well, do not expect all of your thoughts to be positive. When they are not, observe them and learn from them and utilize them to your advantage. Do the same with positive ones.

Peacefulness

The entire purpose of mindfulness practice is to achieve a peaceful state of mind and existence. When you are working on your mindfulness practice, ensure that you include the practice of peace into your daily routines. Be sure to intentionally leave behind anything that is unwholesome for you, whether it be thoughts, passion, or fame. When doing so, you should refrain from completely shedding it in one go. Instead, take your time and shed each layer, not unlike an onion. Let it fall, become peaceful in your new state of existence, and then shed the next layer. This is how personal development works, and it is how you should take on your mindfulness practice. Attempting to accomplish too much too soon will bring about a wide amount of emotional baggage on its own.

In addition to shedding unwholesome experiences, allow yourself the opportunity to truly face problems and learn from them. Spend time thoroughly analyzing and understanding each problem, and then when you are ready let them go. Refrain from dwelling on anything, whether it be happiness, sadness, gain or loss. Instead, simply see it for what it is and then let it go. When you are able to purify your mind in this way, you will be rewarded with peacefulness within' your mind and life. Peacefulness may feel as though it is one of the hardest things to maintain, but it is actually quite simple. Remember the Middle Way, the Four Noble Truths and the Eightfold Path and you will be able to achieve peacefulness in your life in a simplified manner.

Dignity

Dignity is to live within' a state where you earn honor or respect. When you are using dignity in your mindfulness practice, it is important to understand whose honor and respect you are seeking. It is not that of your peers, but rather that of your own. Your entire mindfulness practice and journey of inner self should be around allowing yourself to be able to honor and respect yourself and in turn, you will be honored and respected by others.

When you are practicing dignity, there are things you should consider. You will want to ensure that you harbor wholesome thoughts and that you are not carrying anything that does not serve you. Again, if you are not served by it, let it go. Be clear on all of the sequences and applications within your life and the practices you take on. Practice your mindfulness diligently and consistently, and refrain from doubting yourself or allowing yourself to fall into distracted patterns. When you are being dignified, practice being at ease and compassionate with yourself, others and the world around you. True dignity can be achieved when you are maintaining all of these practices.

When you actively follow and engage in these four principles, you will be able to easily guide your mind through life. At first, you may struggle to do so. However, once you spend more time focusing on each principle and enforcing it in your mind and life, you will discover that it becomes easier. Like with anything, mindfulness and the practices associated with it take the time to nurture and develop. As mentioned, take your time and truly allow yourself to embrace each step so that it makes profound and lasting changes and that you are not left feeling suffering or emotional baggage from the idea that you have failed to achieve mindfulness or peace in your life.

Chapter Summary:

- The four principles will help you achieve mindfulness
- The four principles include: frankness, simplicity, peacefulness, and dignity
- Minimalism assists you in achieving mindfulness in your life
- Mindfulness is an internal and external practice
- Intention is extremely important when it comes to being mindful

Chapter 18: Practical Implementation

Learning how to practically implement mindfulness into your daily life is important. Some of the previous chapters have discussed specific methods, but now you are going to learn about various ways you can incorporate mindfulness into your daily life in some of the most common daily activities that we encounter on a daily basis. The following sections will contain tutorials and tips on how you can become mindful during everyday activities and increase your mindfulness practice.

Seated Meditation

Setting aside intentional time for meditation is important. In the chapter "meditation" you learned a guided body scan that assisted you in checking in with yourself. However, not all meditation requires you to regularly check in with every single body part. Instead, you can be a little more "to the point" per se. In this guided tutorial, you are going to learn how you can meditate without needing to do a total body check in. Instead, you will be able to focus more on your breathing and your sensations associated with the breath and maintain your focus through a counting exercise. This meditation can take significantly less time if you desire, but you can carry it out for as long as you wish. It is a very versatile meditation that brings a great awareness to the body itself, as well as by eliminating stress and dis-ease within the mind and body.

To start, sit in a chair with your feet planted firmly on the floor. You want them to be grounded, so make sure the entire bottoms of your feet are touching the floor. Then, sit with your back tall and straight. Your head should be facing forward, with the top of your head pulled up towards the ceiling so that your spine is elongated. When you are ready, start taking deep breaths in and out. You will want to breathe in through your mouth and out through your nose. Then, when you feel more relaxed, place your hands on your abdomen. Breathe in and count to four. Then, hold it for the count of six. Finally, breathe out for the count of eight. You should do this breathing exercise at least thirty times before you end your meditation session, though you can do it much longer if you desire.

When you notice your awareness start to shift or your thoughts start to wander, simply draw your attention back to your counting and breathing. Then, you can calmly keep your awareness focused can gain all of the benefits from meditating. This simple practice is an excellent way for you to bring yourself back into the room and recompose yourself if you discover that you are starting to wander in your thoughts or are feeling excessively stressed out as a result of your circumstances. When you do this, you gain a greater awareness and wisdom over your own body and you benefit in wonderful ways.

Eating

Eating is a powerful time to become mindful. As you have learned in previous chapters, we tend to be very unaware of our eating habits and as a result, we eat excessive amounts and we do not enjoy the food that we are eating. We tend to make unhealthy food choices or eat excessive amounts of unhealthy food, often eating until the point that we feel sick. When we do this, we will start to feel more and more sick as our body continues to digest the food. If, instead, we were to slow down and enjoy the food, we would likely eat healthier and certainly in lesser portions. You can change your eating practices easily, though it may take some time to become used to the slower eating habits.

In the following description, we are going to consider the practice of eating a chocolate.

Imagine you were to eat chocolate now. There is a chance that you would purchase a chocolate bar, eat it in a few seconds and then be done. You would not experience the chocolate bar or the tastes associated with it and as a result it would be a lot less satisfying than if you were to take your time and enjoy the experience. You may even find that you crave chocolate even more so, or you continue to crave it because you are not satisfied. You may even decide to eat more. At that point, you may begin to feel sick because you have eaten too much.

Instead, take your time and slow down. Experience what it is like to open the chocolate bar wrapper and see the chocolate inside. If you feel inclined to, inhale the smell of the chocolate and enjoy that experience for a few moments before you take your first bite. Then, go ahead and take one bite. Feel what the different ingredients feel like against your teeth, and what the texture is like overall as you chew it. What are the flavors you notice? How does it feel in your mouth? They say that we should chew a bite of food approximately thirty times so that it is ready to be digested by our stomach. You don't necessarily have to chew that long, but chew it until you truly feel satisfied with the flavor you have experienced from the bite. Then, swallow it. What does it taste like now? What is the after taste like? How did the experience overall feel? You should eat each bite like this. You may find that you only eat a couple or that you eat half of the chocolate bar and you put the rest away for a later date. This happens because you have satisfied your craving and desire from less. You have deviated from instant gratification and have entered into a place of sustainable gratification.

You should consider this eating tutorial when you are eating virtually anything. The slower and more intentionally you eat your food, the easier it is to enjoy it and gain more from it. You will feel more satisfied, you will eat healthier portions, and you will be more likely to fuel your body in healthier ways because eating healthier food is typically a more enjoyable sensory experience than eating unhealthy foods. When you do this, you increase the benefit and value you gain from your food.

Driving to Work

Often, we have a set route we drive to work and over the years we become so used to it that the experience itself is something we tend to go on autopilot for. Aside from the fact that this makes us at larger risk for an accident, it is also a time where we tend to vacate our minds and deviate from the present moment. We tend to lose our focus and mindfulness practice during this simple activity. Instead of allowing yourself to go on autopilot, try making your drive to and from work a time where you become more mindful.

Take the time to develop an awareness about your car. What is it like when you drive it? How does it feel on the road? Do you have music playing, and if so what is it? Think about the outside world and what your scenery is like, such as how the sky looks and what your surroundings are. If something has changed, take a moment to notice it, without removing your focus from the road of course. When you are driving, pay attention to the cars around you and refresh your focus and attention. Act like you are driving the route for the first time ever. If you feel too bored by your regular route, consider trying a new route or switching it up occasionally. Doing so can make things fresher and make it easier for you to maintain awareness, attention, and mindfulness when you are driving.

You don't have to restrict your mindful driving practice to the drive to and from work, either. Many of our regular driving routes are affected by this autopilot we tend to go into when we know the road well and feel as though we don't have to focus as much. That is why most accidents happen within' a kilometer of the home. This is a wonderful time to bring your mindfulness practice into place and bring the enjoyment of driving back.

Brushing Your Teeth

Each day you likely brush your teeth at least twice: morning and night. But did you know you can bring your mindfulness skills into this practice, as well? In fact, this is a wonderful time to practice mindfulness. In the morning, it sets the tone for the day. In the evening, it allows you to come back to the present moment before you go to sleep!

You can practice mindfulness easily when brushing your teeth. Start by listening to the water when you turn on the tap to wet your toothbrush. Then focus on what it is like when the toothpaste comes out of the tube onto your brush. How does it fall? What color is it? When you wet the brush again then put it into your mouth, what is the texture of the toothpaste? How does it feel in your mouth and against your teeth? Take the time to notice the textures and sensations as the toothpaste runs through your mouth. If you are using a minty flavored toothpaste, you can likely feel your taste buds changing. You can pay attention to what the bristles feel like against your teeth and gums, and how they feel when you wash off your tongue. When you are done, pay attention to what it feels like to rinse out your mouth. How does the water taste different now that your teeth have been brushed? When you're about to leave the bathroom. take one last moment to notice the aftereffect. How does your mouth feel now? Does it taste better? What is different about your breath?

Brushing your teeth is a wonderful time to bring mindfulness practice into play. You are doing something that for many is a mindless activity. However, there are a great deal of sensations associated with brushing your teeth that can assist you in bringing your awareness and attention back into your body in the present moment. As well, this activity happens to fall at two of the best times to really want to pay attention to bringing mindfulness into your day.

Arriving at and Leaving Work

Work is a place where we often go into autopilot because many people in modern times are not in love with their jobs. Our instant gratification mindsets tend to take over and a job we may have loved when we started quickly becomes a job we dislike or resent. In other times, you may have never liked your job but you feel forced to go because you require money to pay for your life. When you are resentful and unhappy at work, it can be easy to go into autopilot or operate from a mindless place as a means to protect yourself from the unwanted feelings that may arise. What this actually does is cause more emotional baggage.

When you are working, you should especially pay attention to your body and your mind. When you arrive at work, what do you feel like? Are you happy and excited to start your day? Or are you upset and resentful to have to be at work yet again? Either way, you should consider your emotions. If you are upset and resentful, consider using the four principles to assist you in creating a more peaceful mindful practice.

In addition to noticing your emotions, notice external things that you may not be aware of anymore. Focus on what your environment is like, any changes that may have occurred, and anything else that you notice. Pay attention to the lighting, the surroundings, and the physical atmosphere. Take the time to notice who is at your work and acknowledge them if you can.

When you are leaving work, you should take the time to acknowledge what your emotions are like when you go. Are you carrying emotional baggage home with you? If so, now is the time to release your attachment so that you can release your suffering and leave it behind. If not, it is still a good idea to take a moment to gather your thoughts and come out of "work mode" and into "life mode" once again. You should always leave work activities behind whenever possible, as this clears up space in your mind. Bringing home work activities is much like dwelling and can impede your peaceful practices.

Many of us have a tendency to go into mindless autopilot mode around work and work related functions. Whether it's arriving at work, actually working, or leaving work, we have a tendency to "tune out" and we end up carrying around a high amount of emotional baggage as a result. You should consider adding as many mindful practices into your day around work as possible. Doing so will increase your ability to attain inner peace and purification.

Spending Time with Loved Ones

Most people spend time with their loved ones at least once per day. However, many don't actually spend quality time with their loved ones. In the 21st century, we are very consumed by social media, technology, work, and other distractions that can take away from our ability to truly appreciate our time with our loved ones. It is important that you take the time to become mindful about your habit of doing this and do your best to eliminate it. When you are with your loved ones is a wonderful time to work on bringing yourself into the present moment and truly enjoying your time together. Remember, this is impermanent just as everything else in life is, and if you allow yourself to be distracted, you will never be able to get this moment back.

To bring yourself back to the room with your loved ones, take a moment to observe your surroundings once again. Who are your loved ones, and what are they doing? What about them brings you joy? How can you better interact with them and be actively involved in the present moment? Take the time to really bring your appreciation and awareness into the room with you. Put down your phone, turn off the TV, and eliminate other distractions. Take the time to truly engage in some quality time together. You may wish to simply enjoy each other's presence, or you may wish to engage in a conversation or even play board games together or do something else that allows you to bond.

Spending time with loved ones is something we often take for granted, especially when we do it on a daily basis. There is an important quote by Buddha that discusses this, and it is one you should deeply consider when you are too distracted and are not investing enough quality time in your relationship with your loved ones.

"The trouble is, we think we have time." - Buddha

As we learn in Buddhist teachings, the only time we truly have is right now. Everything in the past is gone and everything in the future isn't promised. Life is impermanent, our families are impermanent, everything about the situation you are presently living is impermanent. If you do not take the time to experience it and enjoy it, you will never be able to get it back. It will be lost forever. Time itself is impermanent and we must realize this in order to refrain from taking the ones we love for granted and better enjoy our lives together. Always take the time to invest in mindfulness practice when you are surrounded by loved ones, even if the only one you are surrounded by is your very self.

There are many ways that you can practice mindfulness in your daily life. Many of the areas where mindfulness is best practiced would include activities that we do on a daily basis that are often overlooked. They are the activities we do mindlessly because we are so accustomed to doing them that we no longer realize we are even doing them anymore, or anything associated with doing them. We simply do them as quickly as possible and then move onto the next thing. Our life has been so infused with the go-go-go that we rarely take the time to slow down and pay attention to the present time. When you do this, you infuse mindfulness into your life better and you gain all of the wonderful benefits of inner purification and peace.

Chapter Summary:

- There are many points in your day that you can practice mindfulness
- The activities we tend to be mindless about are the best ones to become mindful about
- Brushing your teeth, driving to work, eating food, and meditating are great times to focus on mindful activities
- Meditating isn't the only way to be mindful
- The more you can practice mindfulness, the easier it is to continue practicing it

Chapter 19: Continuing Your Journey

Our journey together is drawing near the end and it is time for you to gain a strong idea of how you can carry on your mindfulness practices throughout your life. As you may expect, your mindfulness practice does not end when this book does. Many people view mindfulness as a mental diet: they feel as though it is something they only need to practice for a short period of time and then when they achieve results they can stop. The trouble is, just like a diet, if you do not maintain the changes you will revert back to old patterns. Knowing that, you need to be prepared to continue your journey and carry on down the path of mindfulness and practice it for years to come. The rest of your life, in fact.

The thing with mindfulness is that you are never done. There is always another layer inward that you can go, and you will never be complete until you achieve nirvana. And even then, you are not done. That being said, you should continue practicing all of the mindfulness activities that you have learned in previous chapters in this section on a daily basis. The more you practice these, the easier it will be for you to go deeper inward and experience mindfulness on a more powerful basis. Practicing mindfulness will make your practice more powerful and as a result, you will find that it is easier to be mindful on a more regular basis. In fact, you may reach a point where you are mindful at least 90% of the time. This is normal and is also completely achievable if you are not already there.

A large part of mindfulness is simply practicing on a moment-to-moment basis. You want to always be asking yourself the right questions to keep your awareness and attention in the present moment. You always want to ensure that you are not taking time for granted and that you are not becoming too focused on the mind or the body. Rather, you want to maintain a balanced mindful awareness over the mind, body, spirit and environment. In doing so you will make it easier for yourself to stay present and therefore gain the most out of every practice.

Journaling is a great thing to do during the development of your mindful practice and maintains a wonderful activity to continue doing as it allows you to keep a catalog of your thoughts and experiences. You can pay attention to what has worked and what doesn't, you can materialize your thoughts to eliminate them from your mind if that works for you, and you can watch yourself grow as you continue to develop. When you look back through your journals, you will be able to see how far you have truly come and how far you have left to go. It is a great opportunity to become clear with yourself over what you have completed and what you would like to complete. In a way, it is another form of meditating as it allows you to sit with your thoughts for a period of time.

There are other ways that you can infuse your life with mindfulness, and you may wish to include these in your life in some way or form in time. Doing so will assist you in deepening your learnings of mindfulness and the benefit you gain from it. They include yoga, walking, lighting candles and watching them, taking regular breaks, listening, and focusing on your breath. For the last one, you were guided on a meditation on how you can focus on your breath more intently. However, you do not need to completely meditate in order to do so. Instead, you can take a moment here and there to just check in with your breath and see how it is doing. Intentionally practice your 4-6-8 breathing technique and let yourself relax for a moment. Then, go back to your daily activities. By doing this mini-break, you do not have to actually withdraw from any activities. It is something you can do amidst everything else.

One of the biggest things you should think about now and forevermore is that mindfulness is something you can do in your life. It is a lifestyle change you must make and you will continue making it, but it is something you can do. Many people struggle to maintain mindfulness or "achieve" it because it is simply not achievable. It is something you are constantly working on. It can be common to feel somewhat intimidated by it or as though you may not be able to do it, but the truth is everyone can and everyone should.

You do not have to be a Buddhist to learn about mindfulness and practice it; however, the Buddhist teachings are incredible for learning more about the practice of mindfulness and how it can benefit you. You may wish to carry on and learn more about Buddhism so that you can go even deeper into your mindfulness teachings. Or, you may be drawn in a different direction. Either way is completely fine. As long as you are doing what feels right for you, you can't go wrong.

In this book, you have learned several concepts that are powerful in guiding you through your mindful practice. You should continue to consider them and practice them on a regular basis. The Four Noble Truths, the Eightfold Path, the Five Aggregates, the Four

Principles, the Middle Way, the Three Poisons, the Four Marks of Existence, Karma and Vipaka and the Five Precepts are all powerful concepts that can teach you a great deal about your mindfulness practice. If you haven't already spent time on each one and learning about how they affect and influence your life, you should do so now. Take the time to develop an awareness of each concept and how it can influence your life. Take the time to realize where you could use these practices, or where they are affecting you, and then do the necessary work to eliminate the effects of them.

The most important thing is that you continue on. You should keep practicing each day, and each moment whenever possible. Doing this will drive you deeper into your mindful practice and deeper into yourself. You will gain more clarity, more wisdom, and more inner power as a result. You will be able to develop inner purification and peace, a sustainable gratitude and more happiness due to less suffering. Ultimately, as long as you continue practicing your mindfulness strategies in your everyday life, you will lead a life that is more enjoyable. The practice of mindfulness is one that people often overlook, but it is one that is most necessary. In an age where everything is rushed and instant gratification is the driving factor for virtually everything, we need mindfulness now more than ever.

Chapter Summary:

- You can continue your mindfulness practice with the skills you learned previously
- Exercise such as yoga and walking is a great way to stay mindful
- You should take frequent breaks and pay attention to your inner world
- Mindfulness is a balance you practice from moment to moment, you cannot "achieve" it; instead, you experience it
- You should take the time to look deeper into each of the concepts taught previously and recognize how they influence and affect your life
- Journaling is a powerful tool when becoming mindful and growing your practice

Conclusion

We have come to the end of the book and you have learned a lot of powerful information on mindfulness practices. As you have learned, the Buddha was very deep into mindfulness and a great deal of the Buddhist teachings are surrounding teachings of the mind. As we are mental beings, it is important that we learn to regard the importance of our mind and the importance of being able to understand and control it. Mindfulness is a powerful way for you to be able to do that.

There are many ways to achieve mindfulness, but the first is to understand the mind and what mindfulness is. The many teachings of the Buddha allow you to learn wisdom around the mind and the way it works, which ultimately gives you the important tools and keys required in learning to control the mind itself. In many instances, the first step of controlling the mind is letting go of control. Meditation is a common and powerful practice that allows you to learn this and then carry on your way.

The Four Noble Truths of Buddhism are arguably some of the most profound and important teachings for you to learn. Whether or not you desire to be Buddhist, you can learn a great deal from these. You may recall that they are: suffering exists, suffering exists because of attachment, suffering ceases when attachment to desires ceases, and freedom can be achieved through the Eightfold Path. When you consider these Noble Rules, you can then apply them to life in order to cease your suffering and increase your inner purification and peace. The rest of the Buddhist teachings work together with these Noble Rules to assist you in detaching from your attachments and ending the suffering.

There are many ways in which modern society suffers. We have a tendency to be largely driven by instant gratification which, ironically, leads to a great deal of suffering on an individual basis and as a society. Many people realize this and believe that industries and corporations are to blame for the massive suffering. The truth is, they are not. Industries, corporations, and other parts of the consumerist society are proof that we are doing what humans should do. They are proof that we are exercising our minds and our ability to expand. However, when we do not have a healthy interaction with this industry, we eliminate our ability to gain benefit and value from it. Knowing that, it is important that we develop healthy relationships with our consumerism and instant gratification-driven tendencies.

Another equally important teaching to consider is the Middle Way. The Middle Way is a wonderful guiding factor when it comes to leading your life. It allows you to understand that everything can be done, only in moderation. You should never restrict yourself from doing anything, but you should also refrain from doing it excessively. Instead, you should do things in moderation. Do them enough to feel satisfied or to meet a need, nothing more and nothing less. When you lead life by the Middle Way, you preserve yourself from the suffering that comes from being extremely one way or another. You allow yourself to experience all that life has to offer without subjecting yourself to the suffering it has the ability to bring.

Finally, you also need to pay close attention to impermanence. A great deal of suffering that we experience as a modern society is caused by our attachment to the belief that things will always be as they are. We forget to realize that emotions, situations, people, time, and objects are impermanent. Everything we encounter is impermanent. You will not be able to keep anything forever, and eventually, everything goes away. Even you will go away, one day. You should use this to encourage yourself to grow your mindfulness practice each moment and do your best to always stay present in the moment. This gives you the opportunity to truly enjoy all that life has to offer, whether it feels good or not.

You should never run away from experiences, as this builds up emotional baggage. When you run from suffering, you create more suffering. Always be frank and face the reality you are living. Be honest and open, and be welcoming toward criticism as you never know what it may provide you with. When you do, you will almost always great wisdom and awareness into yourself and your life. In one way or another, it will assist you in your growth.

I hope that this helps you when it comes to being able to develop your own mindfulness practice. Hence, you should be able to learn greater insight into your mind and its functions and how you can be at oneness with your mind. We are mental beings and our minds are vital in our existence, so it is important that we learn to understand them and work with them. In modern society, it is common to overlook the mind, but it is not wise. In doing so, you create ignorance and you lead a life that is void of any meaning or purpose.

The next step is for you to take the time to truly and deeply understand the practices you have learned and take the time to become mindful about how they influence or affect you. Understand why they are important and where they are important in your life and what they mean to you. When you do, you can learn how to use that knowledge to further increase your inner peace and purification. As a result, you will likely lead a happier life overall.

You should take the time to meditate on a regular basis, as it is one of the single most important mindfulness practices and therefore it is something you must focus on. You do not necessarily have to sit down and close your eyes to meditate. Instead, you can bring your awareness to your body, the sensations you are feeling, and your breath. In doing so, you will enter a state that allows you to work with your intrinsic mind and it will enable you to further develop your inner world. Thus, your mental and emotional states will become much more balanced and stabilized.

If you enjoyed this book, I hope that you will please take the time to review it on Amazon Kindle. Your honest feedback would be greatly appreciated.

Thank you, and best of luck in your practice!

42917819R00112